FAST FACTS FOR THE CLINICAL NURSE MANAGER

Managing a Changing Workplace in a Nutshell

About the Author

Barbara J. Fry, RN, BN, MEd (adult), is President of Workplace Dynamix, Inc., an active member of the College of Registered Nurses in Nova Scotia, and a Professional Keynote Speaker and Facilitator. She received a BN and Diploma in Teaching in Schools of Nursing from Dalhousie University, Halifax, NS (Canada), a Change Management Certificate from Queen's Univ (1997), and a Master of Adult Education from St. Francis Xavier University (2003). Her master's thesis was "Facilitating Workplace Relational Learning: The Intersection of Power, Caring, and Quality of Work Life." As a former staff nurse, nursing instructor, and nurse manager (for 16 years), she "inspired a climate of personal excellence and professional competence in the workplace." Drawing on her experience as a nurse manager, healthy workplace relationship consultant, professional speaker, and adult educator, Fry shares her wealth of knowledge and "strategies that work" in today's changing healthcare workplace. She provides leadership in improving quality of work life and facilitates individual and group leadership and accountability for creating healthy workplace relationships. As a powerful, humorous, and inspiring speaker she was the Closing Keynote Speaker for the Canadian Nurses Association's 100th Birthday Celebration Conference (2008). Today, Fry continues to advocate and facilitate professionalism in nursing practice and promoting healthy workplace relationships. She is a frequently requested presenter and facilitator in both provincial and national nursing associations.

FAST FACTS FOR THE CLINICAL NURSE MANAGER

Managing a Changing Workplace in a Nutshell

Barbara Fry, RN, BN, MEd (adult)

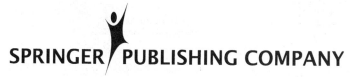

SPRINGER PUBLISHING COMPANY

New York

Springer Publishing Company, LLC
11 West 42nd Street
New York, NY 10036
www.springerpub.com

Acquisitions Editor: Allan Graubard
Production Editor: Barbara A. Chernow
Cover Design: David Levy
Composition: Agnews, inc.

E-book ISBN: 978-0-8261-2569-9

12 13/5 4 3

The author and the publisher of this Work have made every effort to use sources believed to be reliable to provide information that is accurate and compatible with the standards generally accepted at the time of publication. Because medical science is continually advancing, our knowledge base continues to expand. Therefore, as new information becomes available, changes in procedures become necessary. We recommend that the reader always consult current research and specific institutional policies before performing any clinical procedure. The author and publisher shall not be liable for any special, consequential, or exemplary damages resulting, in whole or in part, from the readers' use of, or reliance on, the information contained in this book. The publisher has no responsibility for the persistence or accuracy of URLs for external or third-party Internet Web sites referred to in this publication and does not guarantee that any content on such Web sites is, or will remain, accurate or appropriate.

Library of Congress Cataloging-in-Publication Data

Farquharson Fry, Barbara, 1948–
    Fast facts for the clinical nurse manager : managing a changing workplace in a nutshell / Barbara Fry.
      p. ; cm.
    Includes bibliographical references and index.
    ISBN 978-0-8261-2568-2 (alk. paper)
    1. Nurse administrators—Handbooks, manuals, etc.   I. Title.
    [DNLM: 1. Nursing, Supervisory.   2. Personnel Management. WY 105 F238f 2010]
    RT89.F37   2010
    362.17'3068—dc22
                                                                        2009054128

Printed in the United States of America by Hamilton Printing

Contents

Part III: Staff Gone Wild?
Managing Your Cast of Characters

Part IV: Predicting Your Workplace Future:
Create It! Manage It! Love It!

Preface

Are you and your staff members merely surviving in your workplace or are you thriving? Do you find yourself resolving to start each day reading those nurse management articles and books piled on the corner of your bedside table? Do you have an uneasy feeling that the way you managed two, five, or ten years ago no longer seems to be working as well as it used to? And, despite your best intentions to take better care of yourself, do you find that there is just never enough time for you?

If you answered yes to any of these questions, then there is good news and better news. The good news is that you are not alone. The better news is that this book, *Fast Facts for the Clinical Nurse Manager: Managing a Changing Workplace in a Nutshell,* will give you quick access to insights, strategies, and tools for resolving some of today's most challenging issues for nurse managers.

BACKGROUND

Several years ago, at a time when our world of healthcare first was propelled into an unending cycle of change, I was an experienced nurse manager working in psychiatric/mental health nursing. Following the merger of two hospitals, managers struggled to do more with less in a hostile economic climate dominated by restructuring, reengineering, downsizing and the aggressive introduction of cutbacks and technological change. Declarations of "Manage your budgets or we will find someone who will" fueled the fires of clinical rationalizations, fiscal restraint, and hospital closures, leaving an organizational battlefield littered with the emotional debris of the laid off, downsized, and disenfranchised. In its place, a culture of "survivors" emerged, fearfully awaiting the next round of job cuts and assuming a "safe" mode by keeping their heads down and their "mouths shut."

Nurse managers and senior leadership positions were annihilated at an alarming rate and staff was moved about like pawns on a chessboard. Those managers who kept their jobs were at a loss as to how to manage staff members' growing sense of fear, anger, powerlessness, and disrespect, while providing care to their patients. Rising acuity levels and rapid turnover in patients compounded the stress in the workplace, resulting in deteriorating quality of worklife, increasing use of staff sick time, interpersonal conflict among nurses, and slow burning frustration with a system that no longer seemed to care.

It was during this time that I became what I had most feared—a casualty of organizational change. I lost my job as nurse manager. Faced with answering the question "Now what?" and a situation over which I had no control, I realized that I had the control and the power to choose my attitude in response to what had just happened. Exerting that power would determine the quality of my future.

I was in my late forties and was attempting to embark on a personal journey of transformation inspired by Peter Drucker, a business management theorist and author, who once said, "The best way to predict the future is to create it." Suddenly, through circumstances beyond my control, I was facing my future. As I reflected on the aspects of my life, I asked myself what was important in my personal life and my life as a nurse? As a nurse manager, I knew that I disliked budgeting and staffing (anything to do with numbers), but was inspired by the countless opportunities nurse managers have to impact the professional lives of nursing staff and the resultant effect on the quality of patient/client care. Creating and managing an environment where nurses would want to work, feel proud about being a nurse, and do what they loved was in my mind the ultimate role of today's nurse managers. I knew that none of these outcomes were a reality for most staff and their managers because amid this organizational chaos they were suffering in ways that we had never seen or experienced. My conclusion was that these nurses and their managers needed a nurse!

The next day I met with the Vice-President of Acute Care with a proposal I had written for a new role that would support the 2,300 nursing staff in the organization. I pointed out that millions of dollars were being spent on sick time; staff morale was at an all time low, and recruitment and retention strategies were being challenged. Professional practice was on a slippery slope, as in-fighting and territorial battles erupted among nurses when they turned on one another in frustration as they struggled to survive in their workplaces. Managers needed help in managing the behaviors and the situations that were now emerging and negatively impacting the quality of patient care.

With the VP's enthusiastic support the proposal was accepted, a new role for the organization was born, and I was launched into a unique career. I would be available to staff and nurse managers on a 24-hour basis to assist them in managing change, improving their quality of worklife, and facilitating the creation of healthy workplaces where nurses would want to work. My key messages were, "The world is changing and so must we; we must learn new ways of being, grow, and change the way we work together and how we relate to one another; and regain our focus on professional nursing practice."

Within six years, and eventually working corporate-wide, I sought academic validity of my work by researching the process and completing a master's degree in adult education at St Francis Xavier University in Nova Scotia, Canada.

ORGANIZATION

Part I addresses the need for nurse managers to change how they manage and lead in a changing practice setting. Chapter 1 introduces evolving leadership and managerial practices. In Chapter 2, nurse managers learn the importance of becoming more political within their organizations. Chapter 3 discusses the new competencies that are on the horizon and how to help staff name and prepare to incorporate these into their practice.

Part II discusses the new reality that change is a constant and will impact everyone. To that end, nurse managers must be prepared both personally and professionally. Thus, Chapter 4 discusses the aura of uncertainty that lurks in the corners of every workplace and how to help staff manage it. Chapter 5 addresses the multigenerational workplace by deemphasizing generational differences. Chapter 6 analyzes a number of theories and literature describing the process of organizational change. In Chapter 7, the reader learns what happens when a way of being ends, how that impacts staff, and what can be done to help them let go of the past. Then, Chapter 8 describes the chaos and confusion that can erupt when staff are caught in the middle between the old way and the new. Finally, Chapter 9 points the learning compass to the new way of being.

Part III describes different situations and types of people with whom nurse manager must deal. Chapter 10 highlights resistance as a normal part of change and discusses how to manage it. Attitude is the theme of Chapter 11, which reinforces that each of us has the power to choose the attitude that will impact quality of worklife. Chapter 12 addresses one of the toughest challenges nurse managers face—dealing with the toxic impact of negative behaviors. Finally, Chapter 13 ramps up the previous chapter by tackling the difficult subject of the workplace bully and what to do when there is one on staff.

Part IV discusses the quality of the nurse manager's workplace future and how managers have the power to create, shape, and influence the direction. Chapter 14 describes the importance of work-life balance. Chapter 15 identifies the need for a practice setting mission, vision, and values. In Chapter 16, the focus is on staff meetings as vehicles for transformation. Then, Chapter 17 reveals why nurse managers and staff members need a visible presence beyond the confines of their practice setting.

Part V summarizes the main points of the text, with Chapter 18 listing the concepts and actions that can give managers a jump start on how to begin to create a place where staff will want to work.

DISCUSSION GUIDES

The discussion guides can be modified to fit the needs of the staff and are meant to facilitate discussion using small and large group formats.

SUMMARY

Today, in my own business as a workplace relationship facilitator, professional speaker, and consultant, I continue to work in both businesses and healthcare sectors assisting managers and their staffs to thrive by seeking healthy strategies for responding to their changing workplace.

Fast Facts for Nurse Managers: Managing a Changing Workplace in a Nutshell is a culmination of personal transformation and experience working with nurses and nurse managers across Canada and in the UK. This book shares insights, practical tips, and a few chuckles about FAQ's, issues, and situations in which so many nurse managers and staff find themselves in their daily struggles in a changing workplace.

Fast Facts will help you learn effective ways for creating, managing, leading, and thriving in a place where nurses and others will want to work. My hope is that you will find this *Fast Facts* book helpful as a tool to accomplish three goals:

1. To become more comfortable with and even welcome change.
2. To try out a few "new" competencies in your practice as a nurse manager, such as risk taking, innovation, flexibility, and creativity, that will ease yours and your staff's adaptation to our changing world of work.
3. To develop a measure of confidence as you move forward with a management style that reflects a "new way of being."

Most of all, if this book inspires you to thrive in your changing workplace, then I will have done my job!

Acknowledgments

To the thousands of nurses I have spoken to or facilitated relational learning workshops with—I am eternally grateful for their trust, candor, and optimism, as they set about to learn new ways of being. I would also like to acknowledge and thank them for their laughter and their spirit. Many colleagues have encouraged me to continue my work and supported me along the way. I especially would like to thank the many nurse managers who helped give me my wings and Chris Power, former VP of Acute Care and executive sponsor, who took a leap of faith in supporting the creation of this innovative and unique position many years ago. Thank you my dear colleagues and friends for your advice, support, and laughter: Paula Dembeck, Charmaine McDonald, Anne Fraser, Laurette Burch, Barb Oake, Krista Connell, and D. Dorothy Lander. A big thanks goes to my parents, Ken and Jean Farquharson, who taught me the artful use of intuitive humor in conversations. Finally, I could not have taken this entire journey without the support of my loving husband Peter, who encouraged and supported me in every way to do the work I felt I was born to do.

Part I

The Bottom Line

Managing What Lies Beneath

Chapter 1

The Buck Stops Here

Managing Professional Practice

INTRODUCTION

This chapter reinforces your ultimate accountability as the nurse manager to ensure that professional nursing practice is alive and well in your workplace. It also serves to remind you that despite the heavy demands of managing day-to-day operations, nurse managers must keep a pulse on practice that is evidenced based and guided by Standards of Professional Practice and the Code of Ethics.

In this chapter, you will learn:

1. The nurse manager's accountabilities and responsibilities for leading professional practice environments in a rapidly changing healthcare system.
2. Specific strategies for demonstrating leadership and "walking the talk" about professional practice in the workplace.

TOWARD A NEW WAY OF BEING

The role of today's nurse managers is a work in progress that is evolving from a role once known as and sadly missed by many, the head nurse. In addition to managing the operations of a particular service, nurse managers are now required to serve as nursing practice leaders, facilitators, coaches, and traffic cops (spending their time directing team members and handling any number of individuals coming at them from all directions). In addition, they must inspire the trust and generate attitudes that promote learning, growth, and change, as well as create an environment in which people want to work. Above all, managers have responsibility for safe and ethical practice in the provision of nursing care. Added to their workloads are patient care crises, committee participation, and the ever-popular "other related duties." Is it any wonder that many question their sanity as they try to juggle "all the balls in the air?"

Many nurse managers have little or no formal preparation for this vital role. Moreover, they receive little organizational support and minimal funding for professional development. Gradually, and thankfully, this situation is changing. A day in the life of a nurse manager usually means 80% of their time is spent on managing operational issues and dealing with the erratic, unexpected, and/or unpredictable incidents (hereafter, fondly referred to as "brushfire management").

24/7 IS NOT ENOUGH TIME

Nurse managers are ultimately professionally accountable and responsible for the quality of care delivered to patients

and clients twenty-four hours a day and seven days a week. However, much of their time is spent away from the practice setting performing "other related duties." How do mangers find the time to ensure that professional nursing practice is alive and well within their service area(s)? All too often, nurse managers reluctantly admit that they do not have enough time to monitor practice because of other demands or because they are not physically present in their clinical settings long enough to know what is really going on. Despite the fact that individual nurses and other healthcare professionals are accountable and responsible for their practice and the fact that clinical support is available from clinical nurse educators, mentors, and nurse specialists, no one but the nurse manager has the authority or professional accountability to manage nursing practice. Bottom line: the buck stops with the nurse manager, who is ultimately responsible for the delivery of quality nursing care. Managers must know and never assume that what is going on at the bedside is done according to the Standards of Professional Practice guidelines and the Code of Ethics.

MANAGING CHANGE TO ENSURE SAFE AND COMPETENT PRACTICE

When significant organizational change challenges the professional practice environment, individuals and teams react. How well they navigate change depends in large part on the culture of the specific unit or service and the broader organization. Professional caring behavior can be influenced positively or negatively by variables that include past experience with change, quality of communication during the change process, workload, physical and psychological well-being of individual staff members, professional autonomy, and nursing leadership.

In situations where change is managed well, staff members are usually motivated to maintain a balance between the tasks and processes of nursing practice AND their mindfulness that accountability is not an option. Professionalism in nursing requires demonstration of behaviors that are consistent with and driven by standards of care and evidenced-based practice.

When change is not managed well, staff members feel powerless, disrespected, and anxious about their future. This uncertainty and anxiety may lead to physical, emotional, and psychological strain that causes staff members to retreat into "survival mode." In an environment that seems to be spinning out of control, with ever-increasing burdens of rising acuity levels, a perceived lack of time, and fewer resources, nurses draw upon their energy reserves and vigorously focus on the tasks related to "getting the job done." By focusing on the tasks or technical aspects of nursing practice and believing that they "don't have time for that other stuff," they risk losing sight of their standards and the evidence-based practice on which their license depends.

When nursing and staff practice fall short of professionalism, nurse managers cannot delay in dealing with the situation. At a time when managers and staff complain about the nurse manager "never being there," this is no easy task. More than ever, nurse managers must be available to make their way back to the bedside or practice-setting environment, if only to ensure that patient/client care and safety are in no way compromised because of a failure to uphold the Standards of Practice.

PROFESSIONAL PRACTICE
STANDARDS CHECK-IN

How current are you with respect to your familiarity with Standards of Practice and the Code of Ethics for staff and nursing leadership? While many nurse managers have a tacit understanding, some will readily admit that professional practice guidelines do not significantly factor into their daily stream of consciousness. If that is the case, this must change. **Regardless of the demands that are placed on you during organizational change, your commitment to maintaining nursing practice according to the Standards and the Code must remain stalwart and at the forefront.**

To do this, you must first give yourself time to reflect on where you are with respect to your own familiarity with the Standards; how you use the Standards to guide your administrative practice; and the degree to which you profile the standards among your staff on a day-to-day basis. It might also be helpful to answer the following questions:

1. To what degree do the Standards of Practice and the Code of Ethics influence our professional practice environment?
2. In what ways do staff members demonstrate evidence of utilization of the Standards of Practice in their everyday practice and therapeutic relationships with patients and clients?
3. How do staff members treat one another professionally, and in what way do they apply the Standards to their collegial/professional relationships?
4. In what ways do the Standards of Practice influence patient/client care communication?

5. How much do the standards factor into creating a respectful workplace and healthy workplace relationships?
6. How much time each day do you allocate to discussing patient care and nursing practice and linking them to the standards of practice?

WHEN STANDARDS OF PRACTICE SIGNIFICANTLY INFLUENCE A PRACTICE SETTING

1. Leading and managing nursing staff will require you at all times to hold staff accountable and responsible for the provision of safe, competent, and ethical nursing practice according to Standards of Practice.
2. Nurse managers will have 24/7 accountability and responsibility for managing and coordinating all professional activities of the nursing staff.
3. Nursing care will be both task and process oriented. Focusing exclusively on tasks denies patients and clients the full benefits of a therapeutic relationship that is foundational to professional nursing practice.
4. Nurses will adhere to and routinely reference their Nursing Standards of Practice and Code of Ethics in their delivery of care.
5. Nurse managers will ensure that their own practice is guided by the Code of Ethics and Standards of Practice for Nurse Leaders.
6. The nurse manager's scope of practice, influence, and communication extends beyond the physical boundaries of the clinical practice setting to include the organization, the community, and beyond.

7. Nurse managers spend regular time in their practice settings communicating face to face with staff to monitor practice and promote trust.
8. Staff members will expect their manager to do what they say they will do.
9. Nurse managers regularly demonstrate coaching, mentoring, and support for the staff's professional development.
10. Nurse managers successfully manage change.
11. Managers and staff are open to doing what is right for their patients in a healing and harmonious environment.

STRATEGIES FOR PROMOTING STANDARDS OF PRACTICE

Clearly Communicate Your Expectations

- It is very important for the staff to know your expectations about professional practice in terms of patient safety, competence, and ethical care. At least once a year, schedule a review of the Standards of Practice and Code of Ethics.
- At the meeting, list on a flip chart no more than six key points describing your definition and expectations of a professional nursing practice environment. Create a conversation around your expectations.
- Describe your expectations of them as staff members and as professionals, as well as your expectations of yourself as their leader.
- Provide staff with a hard copy of your beliefs about professional practice (no more than six bulleted points).
- Ask staff members to respond to what you said: what they liked, what they didn't understand, and any other thoughts they might have.

- Discuss the professional standards that guide nursing leadership.
- Pick one or two standards and begin a conversation, for example, about what accountability in professional nursing practice looks like to patients, peers, and other team members.
- Tell staff about your plans to spend time with each of them to discuss their patient care plans and how the standards influence their practice.

Other Activities to Reinforce Professional Practice Standards

- In nursing rounds, periodically discuss how standards influence a particular nursing intervention.
- Invite a clinical nurse specialist or nurse educator to conduct monthly lunch-and-learn sessions that focus on practice standards.
- Ask staff members to share with others their experience with standards influencing practice.
- Discuss with other nurse managers how they use the standards to reinforce professionalism in practices.

THE BOTTOM LINE IS NOT ABOUT MONEY

Nurse managers can easily be consumed by directing most of their professional energies toward managing the operational aspects of a busy practice setting. There are never enough hours in the day. But when you step back and, with a critical eye, examine the underlying engine that drives the practice setting, much is revealed. What you may see is busy people trying to do the best they can for the patients/clients they serve. But you will also see that much of the business is related to "This is the way we always do things around here," patterns of behavior related to the informal culture, or reactive practice in response to rising acuity levels, rapid turnover of patients/clients, and the bone breaking pressure of a system under siege. In the background lies the all too forgotten guidelines to professional practice that are at risk of extinction in the consciousness of practitioners. As the nurse manager, your job first and foremost is to ensure excellent quality nursing care delivered according to the Standards of Professional and the Code of Ethics. Your second job is to manage the necessary resources for nurses and other clinicians to do their jobs.

Fast facts in a nutshell: summary

- Nurse Managers are accountable and responsible 24/7 for the quality of nursing care delivered in their clinical practice setting.
- Nurse Managers must deal with nursing practices that are inconsistent with the Professional Standards of Practice and the Code of Ethics.

Chapter 2

Power, Politics, and Possibilities

Managing the Art of the Possible

INTRODUCTION

Savvy nurse managers know the importance of becoming comfortable with the "P" words: positive personal and professional power, becoming political, and seeing the possibilities in a changing workplace. The more nurse managers know and use these words to guide their leadership actions, the more influential and successful they will become in facilitating the critical linkages among professional nursing practice, quality of worklife, and organizational success.

In this chapter, you will learn:

1. Attitude is the seat of personal and professional power.
2. How "P" words can transform yours and your staff's professional practice.
3. Strategies to guide your political development using personal and professional power.

"P" WORDS: POSITIVE POWER, POLITICS, AND POSSIBILITIES

In the early days of healthcare restructuring, the battle cry of "lead, follow, or get out of the way" heralded a paradigm shift that resulted in organizational restructuring, revision of work processes and resource allocation. Nurse managers were also challenged to manage their budgets or "or we will find someone who will." In the end, they were left feeling they had few choices. While some bravely decided to "lead" despite being unsure about what this "new" leadership would look like, many fell victim to an overwhelming sense of powerlessness. Hoping to defend themselves against job loss, nurse managers dug into their workplace bunkers, struggled to support their staffs, and turned their attention to survival mode. They focused on their budgets, doing more with less, and maintaining the status quo for fear of "making a career limiting move."

POWER, POLITICS, AND POSSIBILITY PONDERABLES

Even with positional power, many nurse managers continue to feel powerless, "caught in the middle," and "that they have the responsibility without the authority." It is important to try to determine how much power you have in the organization by considering the following:

- How much personal and professional power do you feel you have at this moment? How comfortable are you in sharing power through delegation?

- Are you politically savvy enough to know what is happening beyond the four walls of your unit or organization, to acquire the resources you need to provide safe, ethical, and competent care, and manage complex workplace relationships?
- And, by the way, what is your Possibility Quotient? How excited are you about the possibilities that exist in the evolving world of healthcare?

The nursing literature tells us that nurses tend to shy away from the use of "P" words, especially "power" and "politics." "Power" is regarded as antithetical to "caring." Nurses will substitute "empower" for the word "power" to soften the perception of what may sound offensive to caring ears. And while nurses can readily express their feelings of powerlessness, they struggle with conversations about developing a sense of personal and professional power.

Nurse managers can model the use of positive language that reflects personal and professional power to help staff members move beyond using "soft" language that demeans, minimizes or marginalizes their practice. The manager is the person with the positional power to lead nurses to discover the possibilities that lie within and the capacity to help facilitate their professional transformation.

Fast facts in a nutshell

- Nurses must get comfortable with "P" words.
- These include personal and professional power, politics, and possibilities.

> • Using "P" words to create new conversations can lead to new learning, growing and changing

POWER TO CHOOSE YOUR ATTITUDE

Before you can adequately lead your staff in getting comfortable with personal and professional power, politics, and possibilities in a changing workplace, you must first determine where you fit. To do this, **give yourself the gift of time to reflect on your own quality of worklife, your attitude, and your willingness to change.** Ask yourself the following questions:

• Where are you on the ladder of professional power in your organization?
• Are you feeling powerless in the system, within your peer group, or with your staff?
• Do you believe you have the competencies that demonstrate personal and professional power?

ATTITUDE MATTERS

The following statements can serve as guiding principles for you to embrace as you consider the scope of your personal and professional power as a nurse manager:

1. **The one thing I have power over in my worklife is the attitude I choose in response to change.**

2. No one else is responsible for my attitude.
3. The quality of my worklife future and workplace relationships will largely depend on the attitude I choose.
4. I know that the best way to predict my future is to create it.
5. The only person I can change is me.
6. To successfully manage my changing workplace, I must be willing to learn, grow, and change.
7. Memo to self: For every crisis there is opportunity; there are two sides to every coin; yada, yada, yada!

CHOOSING POWERLESSNESS

What attitude will you choose? If you choose powerlessness:

- You will quickly learn that your behavior will lead to acting powerless.
- You will talk like a victim by whining about almost everything and wondering why others don't realize "how difficult it is for us . . . " or complaining that "I don't know what's going on around here, nobody tells us anything."
- **You may unwittingly give permission to your staff members to become victims as well.** In organizational speak, this is known as the "cascade effect," where behaviors at the top of the organization spill over and get played out in the actions of the frontline staff.

Fast facts in a nutshell

- You have power to choose your attitude (the Devil doesn't make you do it!).
- Attitude is a powerful determinant in quality of work-life.
- There are positives and negatives in every situation; the key is to find and act on the positives.

CHOOSING A POSITIVE PERSONAL AND PROFESSIONAL WAY OF BEING

As the nurse manager, you can be the most positive influence on the staff's ability to adapt to a changing workplace. **When you choose a positive attitude as a personal and professional way of being, you become personally and professionally powerful.** You will not only strengthen your own sense of well-being, you will inspire others to do the same.

TWELVE TERRIFIC STRATEGIES FOR POWERING UP PERSONALLY AND PROFESSIONALLY

Create "AHA!" moments for yourself by reflecting on and admitting that in today's complex healthcare environment you cannot be all things to all people, that you do not have all the answers, and you will do the best possible job within the limitations of your human, fiscal, and personal resources, and that the world will keep on turning. To that end, try the following:

1. **Resolve to embark on a journey of new learning to increase your personal and professional power for leading change in the workplace.** Think about traveling along a metaphoric road that has many side roads: some you will take, others you may not choose, a few may entice you halfway along, others may come to a dead end. Simply turn round and choose another path.
2. Recognize that this journey "is not one more thing you must do." Make it an adventure in self-discovery, and gasp . . . it might even be fun!
3. Start by giving yourself time to reflect. Think about someone you have worked with or currently work with—someone you consider to possess exemplary leadership qualities.
4. Write down these amazing qualities, and think about your own style of managing and leading.
5. Consider the following: What are your strengths? What areas could you improve on? How closely aligned are your qualities with those of the person you most admire?
6. Identify the relationships and situations in the workplace that push your "powerless" buttons.
7. List the situations over which you have no control and immediately put them aside.
8. Create a priority list for dealing with situations over which you have influence and control. Name the issues, and create an action plan.
9. Learn everything you can about managing the power dynamics and relationships across the levels in the organization.

10. Develop a personal learning plan for building on your leadership competencies that will assist you in your journey toward a new way of being.
11. Give yourself permission to try behaviors to see what fits. At first, this may feel uncomfortable to you and others, but stick with it and remind yourself that you cannot be responsible for how others react toward the emerging new you!
12. Lighten up, be kind to yourself, and don't forget to have fun!

POWERING UP POLITICALLY

Political acumen is necessary for nurse managers to secure resources, manage conflict, and build relationships to get the work done and ensure optimum levels of care. Consider these political skills ponderables:

1. How skillful are you in inspiring others?
2. How well do you engage your staff and influence colleagues in considering new possibilities, directions, and policies?
3. How in tune are you with your staff's power dynamics (i.e. RNs, LPNs, and other members of the multidisciplinary team)?
4. How well informed are you about the power dynamics within your organization?
5. How well do you interface with other nonnursing managers and leaders?
6. How good are you at breaking through the "silos" and forging new relationships?
7. How well do you manage conflict?

By turning these ponderables into action steps for new learning, you are well on your journey toward effective management of your changing workplace.

Fast facts in a nutshell

- Women are inherently relational, which makes them well suited for the political arena.
- Nursing practice is about managing professional relationships, so nurses know how to be political. They just don't necessarily recognize or name their actions as such.

A NOTE OF CAUTION: WHEN NURSE MANAGERS HANG OUT WITH STAFF

The power dynamics between nurse managers and staff members is a delicate one. When nurse managers party and socialize with staff on a regular basis, mixed messages are sent. Because the incumbent nurse manager is required to manage performance, evaluate quality of service, and hire and fire, socializing can lead to blurred professional and social boundaries. When a manager's friendship is tossed into the professional relationship mix, the resulting situation has the potential to create relational hardship, workplace tension, accusations of favoritism and unfairness, ambivalence, and uncertainty. Hanging out with staff becomes particularly problematic when the manager has to discipline a staff member who is also a good friend.

There are many reasons why this dynamic develops, but it is usually explained as a means for nurse managers to "get staff to like them." Another reason could be the manager's attempt to reinforce the concept of team, the idea that "we're all in this together." While these strategies may seem to work in the short term, they rarely work in long term. **Bottom line: You cannot be a friend and effectively manage staff.** In a professional practice environment, relationships must be grounded in professional behaviour for both managers and staff. In locations where "everybody knows everybody," particularly in small communities, it is very important to have the conversation with staff about boundaries around professional relationships and how they are to be managed in the workplace.

Fast facts in a nutshell

- Bottom line: You cannot be a friend and effectively manage staff.

MANAGING THE ART OF THE POSSIBLE

In a changing workplace, nurse managers know that curve balls can be thrown at anytime from anywhere! Plans and people come and go, and the only constant is change. Our world of work in healthcare has never been here before. To paraphrase Albert Einstein, we cannot solve today's problems with yesterday's solutions. We have to find new ways of working together, and no template exists to show us how to move forward. To that end, there are only possibilities. Nurse managers and staff must step away from self-limiting comments, such as "We've always done it this way." Instead, ask the question, "What is possible, or what possibilities exist." These types of questions throw the doors wide open to new ways of thinking, working, and being.

Simply asking about possibilities inspires new conversations and stimulates new learning opportunities to facilitate a journey of transformational change! Nurse managers have the power to facilitate self-discovery in each staff member and to inspire the professional power that lies within the staff group. Transformed nursing staff is capable of exceeding performance expectations, creating an environment where people want to work, and demonstrating personal and professional power in their practice. Staff energy is palpable and the possibilities are endless.

Fast facts in a nutshell: summary

- "P" words, such as positive personal and professional power in practice, politics, and possibility, can be the foundation for individual and workplace transformation.
- Facilitating professional power through self-discovery and self-mastery is both a gift and a responsibility of nurse managers.

Chapter 3

Competencies for a Changing Workplace

Managing New Rules and New Roles

INTRODUCTION

Do your staff members cling to old patterns of working just because "we've always done it this way"? This chapter will assist you in facilitating their understanding of and the necessity for all of us to acquire the competencies that help us to adapt to a new world order. As new rules, new roles, and new competencies emerge, each of us must make a choice to move toward a "new way of being," remain the same, or stick our heads in the sand. Will this situation precipitate a personal or professional opportunity? Who knows? The choice is ours to make!

In this chapter, you will learn:

1. The impact of transitioning from the good ol' days to a "new way of being."

2. The key competencies that will positively influence nursing practice in a changing workplace.
3. Strategies to manage the new competencies.

OH! THE TIMES THEY ARE A CHANGIN'

Reinforcing reality is a principle we all learned in psychiatric and mental health nursing. It remains a useful tool for today's nurse managers in helping staff understand the requirement for personal and professional change in order to thrive in today's practice settings. In many cases, organizational changes are being driven by global economic and technological forces. Thus, they are beyond staff control. However, a number of staff members will actually believe that "All this change is the direct result of some the hare-brained scheme, developed by unknown people, sitting in a dark room deliberately planning ways to mess up our lives."

REMEMBERING THE GOOD OL' DAYS

In the past, changes in nursing practice often resulted from internal requirements to improve patient care efficiencies, quality of care, and service delivery. Now, nursing practice is evidence–based, complex, and subject to the influence of drivers that include economics, technology, acuity levels, an aging population and workforce, dwindling human resources, and restructuring. In a world where change is the only constant, **nurses must embrace new competencies, new rules, new roles, new structures, and new opportunities**, whether they like it or not! Your job is to help them understand and manage these requirements.

EXTRA! EXTRA! READ ALL ABOUT IT!
PROFESSIONAL NURSING PRACTICE
IN A STATE OF TRANSITION

Many organizations and professional disciplines are finding themselves caught in the middle of a Clash of the Ages, from the hierarchical mindset and practices of the Industrial Age to the Age of Information and Technology (to be followed by old age for some), and then on into the Age of Creativity. Quite a leap in a matter of a few decades!

Transitioning and adapting to a changing workplace can be particularly challenging for staff who are seniors (born before 1945) and their Baby Boomer colleagues (born between 1945 and 1965), who spent the majority of their worklives in highly structured, top-down, command and control environments.

YOU'VE COME A LONG WAY, BABY!

The nurse manager, formerly head nurse role, has undergone unprecedented change in the last two decades from job titles and descriptions to scopes of management practice. Some may argue that the changes and expectations have "made things worse." Others can barely contain their excitement about the opportunities that come with a position that can potentially influence improvements in service delivery and nursing practice on an individual, organizational, and global level. The following provides a brief glimpse and tongue-in-cheek description of the head nurse role in the good ol' days of the 1960s, 1970s, and 1980s, and concludes with a brief overview of the still-evolving nurse manager role.

A BIRD'S EYE VIEW OF THE GOOD OL' DAYS OF NURSING MANAGEMENT

Many nurses gaze fondly on the past, longing for the stability of seemingly less complex times, when head nurses were always there, answered all questions related to patient care, and ruled their roosts with an authoritarian style of leadership. They were *the* source of all things nursing. They had little power and influence in organization-wide decision-making and their workplace operations and budgets were decentralized and managed by those who had little or no knowledge of the practice setting, and hiring was a function of human resources.

THAT'S NOT MY JOB!

The head nurse's influence could only be extended as far as the job description would allow. These descriptions were prescriptive and numbered with a final category of other related duties tacked on the end. They frequently became a bone of contention between union and management. If staff was asked to do something not listed, the response was likely to be, "That's not in my job description. If you make me do it, I'll grieve!" In the good ol' days, the union would be all over the head nurse like fleas on a dog. The head nurse was silenced.

THE WORKPLACE HOW-TO POLICY AND PROCEDURAL MANUAL: INSTRUMENT OF THE DEVIL?

More than almost anything, policy and procedure manuals influenced practice in the good ol' days. Originally designed to guide safe practice, the manuals soon morphed into a bureaucratic monster that covered every imaginable action that staff might ever have to take. Once dutifully written, their completion heralded, read, and initialed by staff, they were banished to ever-growing bookshelves until called on! Taking on mythic proportions, they quickly became the showcased and dust-covered tomes that many considered to be the "law" in nursing practice. If a staff member was asked to perform a task or procedure that could not be found in the policy and procedure manual, they might be overheard saying, "If it isn't written in the P & P manual; it doesn't exist, and I won't or can't do that!"

THE UNION/MANAGEMENT HARD LINE

In the past, relationships between union and management were more adversarial and inclined to focus less on professional practice and more on wages and job preservation. The workforce was primarily homogenous with respect to gender, ethnicity, and age.

TODAY'S NURSE MANAGERS

Today's nurse managers work in what Vaill (1996) aptly refers to as "white water" workplace environments, where they frequently have operational responsibility for complex multiple practice settings and 24-hour accountability for the delivery of safe, ethical, and competent nursing care. In addition, many are involved at the organizational and community level, participate in special interest groups, and are presenters at national and international conferences.

BYE BYE JOB DESCRIPTIONS?

Written job descriptions cannot possibly cover every aspect of nursing's full scope of practice. Rapid technological changes, delegated medical acts, and changing patient demographics make it difficult to keep job descriptions current. Because of the complexities of the practice environment and patient acuity, staff members must be flexible and do whatever it takes within their scopes of practice to properly care for patients and clients.

POLICY AND PROCEDURE MANUALS: RELICS OF THE PAST?

Nursing staff's overreliance on policy and procedure manuals must slowly go the way of dinosaurs and be replaced by technological resources, critical thinking skills of practitioners, and evidenced-based practice. Because Gen Xer's and

Yer's prefer to use technology-based resources, as opposed to reading manuals, and want to help the environment by "saving the trees," they may add momentum to the creation of accessible, on-line resources.

NURSE MANAGERS AND UNIONS: ADVERSARIES OR COLLABORATORS?

It is all about relationships! Adversarial relationships between unions and management are no longer working. While many staff members from the Senior and Boomer generations were influenced by unions, younger generations are less inclined to feel the need. Responding to this demographic shift, many **union and nursing management relationships are guided less by demands for job security and pay incentives and more by creating collaborative relationships** that are aimed at improving the quality of worklife, healthy workplaces, and professional development opportunities.

Fast facts in a nutshell

- What is hot? New competencies: risk taking, creativity, flexibility, and innovation.
- What is not? Rigid job descriptions, policy and procedure manuals, and command and control leadership styles.
- What's exciting? Collaborative union-management relationships.

NEW COMPETENCIES: RISK–TAKING, INNOVATION, CREATIVITY AND FLEXIBILITY

To lead and manage today's nursing staff, nurse managers need to help staff members reflect on how they can enhance their practice and professional presence by strengthening, incorporating, and reenforcing the "new" competencies. But, here's the rub. **These competencies are not new for nurses.** They are deeply embedded in nurses "daily clinical practice," but are not named as such. Rarely do nurses refer to themselves as innovators, risk takers, creative, or flexible. They are more likely to say, "I am just a nurse."

Risk Taking

Risk taking within the context of clinical practice is not about putting patients at risk. It is about a willingness to change, to try something new, to offer to lead when others refuse and speak out when others choose silence. It is also about stretching beyond our comfort zones and occasionally taking a leap of faith.

Innovation

The word "innovation" is relatively new to everyday clinical practice. It must become second nature to every nurse's practice and be named as such. Typically, nurses do not think of or name their practice as "innovative." Instead, they will dismiss their actions with a, "I just did what I had to do for the well-being of my patient." Managers can help nurses reframe their actions as innovative rather than "ho-hum routine."

Creativity

In the Industrial Age mindset, the word "creativity" was not a normal part of the organizational lexicon. In fact, policies, procedures, and practice were designed to create conformity in an era when creative thinkers were often labeled as "off-the-wall, boat rockers"—and worse. Staff members are now asked to become creative by "thinking out of the box." However, many Seniors and Boomers, scarred by organizational change and haunted by memories of recrimination and putdowns, believe that it is not safe to speak out for fear of once again being labeled, marginalized, or put at risk by making a career limiting move. Creativity can only flourish in a workplace where mistakes are considered opportunities to learn, trust is high, and mutual respect is expected.

Flexibility

Flexibility in assignments and tasks, as well as participation in learning opportunities and processes, can inspire flexibility among nursing staff, strengthen interpersonal relationships, and boost morale. Flexibility in practice settings requires us to do whatever it takes to meet the complex needs of our patients/clients. It is no longer acceptable in practice to snarl, "That's not my job!" Workplaces steeped in informal rules and expectations of conformity to the "way we do things around here," stunt personal and professional growth and deny patients the full benefits of best practice and professional nursing care. A "can do" attitude among staff members promotes patient-centered care and demonstrates flexibility and a willingness to learn, grow, and change.

Fast facts in a nutshell

- The new competencies are risk taking, innovation, creativity, and flexibility.
- These "new competencies" are not new to nurses. They have always been integral to nursing practice; we just never named them as such.

FROM NO NAME TO NEW NAME: TIPS TO HELP STAFF MEMBERS REFRAME THEIR PRACTICE

Nurse managers can inspire staff to build a thriving workplace culture by using contemporary language to reflect nursing practice. It may feel awkward at first, but it will eventually become mainstream. Note the following:

- When you change the language, you change the culture. Try linking the word "research" to "innovative" practice. Instead of saying, "Jane had a good idea," try saying, "Jane was very creative. . . ." Or, instead of saying, "Susie volunteered. . . ." try saying, "Susie demonstrated leadership when she. . . ."

- Help staff members reframe their work. Replace "I'm just a nurse so I don't know" with "As a nurse, I do know that. . . ."
- Talk about collaboration when you talk about "working together."
- The word TEAM has been overworked to the point where staff members' eyes glaze over at its very mention. Try words such as "workgroup, peers, staff group, and colleagues."
- Avoid saying, "*My* staff." This moves them out of the professional context into ownership by you.
- Teach staff members to avoid using the term "girls" when referring to their professional relationships.
- Think about other words that diminish nursing professional practice value in the workplace.
- Model the use of terms to profile professional nursing practice.

Fast facts in a nutshell: summary

- If you want to change the culture of your practice setting, use language that reflects a new way of being, such as relational, respect, innovative, spirit, and honor, when describing desirable behaviors.

Part II

The Here and Now
Managing New Realities

Chapter 4

Anticipating Change

Managing Staff Anxiety, Uncertainty, and Fear

INTRODUCTION

Change is the only constant in healthcare organizations as they adapt to today's realities. Staff nurses face countless challenges as they struggle to provide care in environments fraught with uncertainty. Simply anticipating the next round of changes can set off an undercurrent of staff anxiety and fear throughout their practice settings. Many staff members turn to their nurse manager for answers to questions, even when there may be none. Left unexpressed, fear-based emotions can spread like a malignancy, taking on a life of their own and negatively impacting the quality of worklife and patient care. This chapter will help you to manage and lead staff through that fear, anxiety, and uncertainty about the future.

In this chapter, you will learn:

1. The importance of identifying change-induced anxiety and fear of the unknown in yourself and your staff
2. Strategies for managing anxiety and fear in the workplace.

ANXIETY, UNCERTAINTY AND FEAR IN A CHANGING WORKPLACE

Anxiety and fear in the workplace shrouded in a climate of uncertainty are heightened during significant organizational change. The constant fear of job loss poses the greatest threat to the emotional well-being of most leaders and staff. At such a time, nurse managers bear several burdens. In addition to managing the operational aspects of a practice setting, **nurse managers must be adept at helping staff manage emotional responses to the threat of change**, as well as managing their own fears.

When organizational change requires cost-cutting and efficiency measures, nurse managers may be under extraordinary pressure to do more with less, particularly since their overall performance is being judged on whether they achieve the bottom line. Often caught between "a rock and a hard place," they too may fall victim to anxiety, uncertainty, fear, and feelings of self-doubt. Many may wonder, "How do I support my staff when I am feeling so vulnerable?" If you are feeling this way, you need to recognize and acknowledge it. Otherwise, you cannot help your staff manage change. You must make and take time to reflect on your workplace situation, name your feelings, and plan how you will manage them.

Fast facts in a nutshell

- Many nurse managers and their staffs may have to unlearn previous coping behaviors and learn new ones to adapt to a changing workplace.
- Nurse managers must go first in modeling a new way of being!

GO AHEAD, EXPRESS YOURSELF!

When faced with anything new, it is normal to experience a psychological reaction. However, when butterflies take up permanent residence in your stomach and fear at work prevents you from doing your job well and begins to negatively impact your private life, you must take actions to deal with these powerful emotions.

Naming our feelings can be difficult for nurses because many were taught not to express their feelings while providing patient care. Now that "the soft or people issues" are becoming integral to organizational success, **nurses will have to unlearn the imposed stoicism of "Never express your feelings in front of a patient or at work."** Many will have to embark on a new learning curve to learn to express (at least to themselves) what they are feeling, name it, and deal with it.

Both large- and small-scale organizational change evokes a variety of responses among staff. These **responses range from indifference to the ripple of mild concern to the outright devastation of a tsunami!** The extent of anxiety and fear among staff members in your workplace depends on a number of variables including:

1. The magnitude of change (i.e., unit closure, relocation, or the presence of a new nurse manager).
2. The organizational and workplace culture.
3. How well the organization handled change in the past.
4. What change means to individuals and their personal circumstances.
5. The individual and staff's capacity to cope.
6. The support that staff members perceive and receive from senior leadership and their nurse manager.

Fast facts in a nutshell

- The emotional impact of organizational change can be made better or worse depending on the nurse manager's ability to listen carefully, "read" staff accurately, and sensitively respond to staff needs.
- Listening and responding to what staff is not saying is vitally important.

THEY NEED TO JUST GET ON WITH IT, RIGHT?

Some senior leaders and nurse managers believe that when changes are required of staff, "they should just get on with it." Lessons from the days of reengineering tell us that **if we do not attend to the emotional needs of staff, the bottom line will never be achieved.** When needs remain unmet, they turn into behaviors characterized by anger, frustration, sabotage, and disengagement. While a "stiff-upper-lip" approach may work for some staff in the short term, in all probability it will lead to emotions being rerouted underground only to surface in behaviors that may lead to poor quality of care, low morale, and increasing use of sick time.

THE IMPORTANCE OF FILLING IN THE BLANKS

In situations where staff members do not understand the need for change or feel unheard when they ask questions, the conditions become ripe for misinformation. **If staff members meet with silence or receive an inadequate or dismissive response to a question, they will fill in the blanks with an answer of their own.** This attempt to "plug the information gap" primes the pump for the rumor mill wheel to start churning out a cascade of rumors, hearsay, and mayhem!

YOU CAN'T MAKE STAFF "BUY INTO" CHANGE

During significant organizational change, it is important for nurse managers to know that no matter what the "party line" or the reason given for a specific change, "This change will create a seamless continuum of care for our patients . . . ," the question on the minds of most staff members will likely be, "What's in it for me? How will this change mess up my life? Will this change really make a difference?" **Generally, staff members keep these questions to themselves and dutifully nod at the leader's pronouncement.** Leaders look out at the sea of bobbleheads convinced that they have "staff buy in."

They could not be further from the truth. When organizational trust is at an all time low, leaders need to think about the level of trust in their organization before they can expect staff to endorse proposed changes.

IT'S A MATTER OF TRUST

The worst thing any leader can say with respect to change is, "Trust me. This will result in significant improvement in. . . ." The second worst thing is to say is, "We need your buy in." When you ask staff to "buy into" change or when you are directed to "get their buy in," you unwittingly set up a dialogue or resistance in staff members' heads. "Buy in" implies that someone may be trying to get you to do something that you otherwise might not want to do. It is reminiscent to many of a conversation one might have with a car salesperson who wants you to buy a wreck! **Buy in is not the issue; trust is.**

Fast facts in a nutshell

- Staff members are more like to engage in change when they have timely and accurate information, open conversations, feel heard, and trust the messenger.

Even in areas not directly affected by change, most staff members do not trust a leader's reassurances that "things will be okay" and that they will be "safe" or unaffected by change. Many will experience deep fear or anxiety. Their lack of trust in relation to possible job loss is usually reflected in the statement, "If it can happen to them, it could happen to us." Nurse managers can help staff manage this fear and bridge the trust gap.

Building organizational and leadership trust is a slow and complex process, in which actions speak louder than words. However, staff members are generally more willing to trust their Nurse manager as a reliable source of information until something happens to break that trust. When nurses trust their manager, they feel comfortable in expressing their opinions, feel heard and respected, and are more willing to listen to feedback about their performances and go where they are led.

When staff members truly "get the reason" for a particular change, they are more likely to engage in activities that support the change initiatives, become involved in implementation, and see themselves as a part of the whole rather than isolated from the rest of the organization. Anxiety diminishes, attention shifts to "we, not me," and feelings go from surviving to thriving.

CALMING THE TEMPEST IN THE TEAPOT: MINIMIZING STAFF FEAR AND ANXIETY

Nurse managers have an important role to play in creating safe havens for weathering the storms of organizational change and the aftermath. The following actions go a long way in helping nursing staff manage both large and small scale change.

1. **Communicate, communicate, and communicate.** Use two to three different media to communicate information about

change in the workplace. Knowing that staff members differ in their preferences for modes of communication, you can hopefully avoid the ever-favorite response, "Nobody ever tells us anything." Some like written memos, while others prefer face-to-face communication. Effective communication provides an opportunity to be creative. For example, for staff under the age of thirty, why not try text messaging them? But, be careful with e-mails. When emotional content is part of or is implied in the message, scrap it

2. **Establish a mechanism for regular communication updates to keep staff informed.** The more staff members feel a part of the information loop, the more likely they are to continue to support change initiatives, feel respected, and trust in you as their manager.

3. **Create opportunities for staff members to provide feedback on what they heard.** Ask staff members what they like about what they heard and what they are not clear about. You might also ask for comments or suggestions.

4. **Reinforce reality.** Help staff members to understand that proposed changes will happen with or without their permission. That being said, there may be opportunities for staff input into how changes are implemented. It is helpful for staff to know what is negotiable and what is not.

5. **Manage "I heard it through the grapevine!"** Ensure that communication is accurate and timely. Information that travels through the organizational grapevine travels at the speed of light and, if false, can create unnecessary pain and anxiety. Many rely on grapevine communication without regard for accuracy. Nurse managers can help guide staff to seek out reputable sources and encourage clarification of misleading information. When someone makes the state-

ment, "I heard that . . . ," invite that person or offer to "check out" the information for accuracy.

6. **Never say, "I can't talk about that right now"** when responding to a question from a staff member. Nothing will ignite suspicion and generate anxiety faster than a dismissive statement. Staff will immediately begin to speculate as to why you cannot say anything and, in no time at all, fill in the information void. If you do not know the answer to a question, simply say, "I don't have an answer for you at this time but I promise as soon as I find out anything I will let you know." Or try, "I don't have the information you are looking for but I will find out what I can and get back to you." If at the end of the week you still do not have the information, tell them that and assure them that you are still trying.

7. **Staff can handle the whole truth better than half truths.** Openness and transparency communicate respect and build trust no matter what the news.

Fast facts in a nutshell

- You can never communicate too much during times of change.
- Communication Rule: Get the right message to the right person at the right time.

THAT FUZZY STUFF MATTERS

Managing anxiety, fear, and uncertainty among staff is first a matter of understanding your own reactions to change, naming what you are feeling, dealing with those feelings and then tuning into what your staff may be feeling. The steps that nurse managers can take to help staff members manage their anxieties and fears should be premised on trust, mutual respect, and principles of open and transparent communication delivered in an environment of compassion and empathy.

Fast facts in a nutshell: summary

- Ignoring the feelings of staff may slow the progress of change
- Managing feelings in response to change builds trust between the manager and staff and hastens staff's engagement in the change process.

Chapter 5

Got Gap?

Managing the Multigenerational Workplace

INTRODUCTION

The complexities of today's changing world of work become more interesting with the presence of at least 4 generations in the workplace. Managing, a mixture of values, life experiences, and work ethics can either be a nightmare or a dream for nurse managers. When nurse managers are guided by the principle and require "respect for all," they lay the foundation for healthy workplace relationships regardless of the generational mix.

In this chapter, you will learn:

1. The key characteristics of the four main cohorts of generations in the workplace: Seniors, Boomers, Generation Xers, and Generation Yers.
2. What each generation values, needs, and is motivated by.
3. Strategies for managing the multigenerations.

With differing life experiences, values, and expectations about work, **the potential for intergenerational conflict in many of today's workplaces is very real.** Staff members can get caught up sniping at one another with such generational comments as, "These young nurses don't know anything!," or "Why don't those old ducks just retire and make room for me!" The biggest sources of contention among the different generations lie in their perceptions of work ethics, the use of technology, and "the way things used to be done around here." While generation bashing happens within each cohort, the Boomers need to think twice before they bash the Gen Xers and Yers. Why? Because the Boomers produced them! Nurse managers who facilitate intergenerational understanding help decrease interpersonal tension and improve the quality of workplace relationships.

Fast facts in a nutshell

- Time spent on generation bashing depletes staff energy, redirects focus away from patient care, and flies in the face of the Standards of Practice that require nurses to support one another in practice.

KNOW YOUR GENERATIONAL MIX

Nurse managers should at least have a basic understanding of what makes each generation tick and clearly articulated expectations about how staff members treat one another. With the plethora of available research on the multigenerational workplace, it is easy to become overwhelmed with information about how to manage them. The American Psychiatric Nurses Association's statement of Philosophical Beliefs of Psychiatric Nursing Practice offers basic principles that capture the essence of what we all require in our relationships at work regardless of the generation we represent. Adapted from that source, these beliefs provide a nice framework to guide nurse manager's actions to promote healthy intergenerational relationships.

FOR YOUR CONSIDERATION: EXCELLENT PRINCIPLES TO LIVE BY

Try using and referring to these principles adapted from American Psychiatric Nursing Association to guide relationships among all staff members, as well as your relationship with them.

- The need for respect is universal among human beings.
- All individual have intrinsic worth and dignity.
- Every individual has the potential to change.
- All behavior is purposeful and meaningful.

Taking each one of the above can be a framework for how the generations work together. Facilitating staff discussions about what each of these statements would look like in their peer group relationships would be inspiring to say the least.

Fast facts in a nutshell

- Regardless of generation, all individuals have a basic need to be treated with dignity and respect.
- Nurse managers must lead and facilitate this process among staff.

INTERESTING TIDBITS ABOUT THE GENERATIONS

The following time span of years attributed to each generation are not carved in stone. Some individuals possess characteristics from both groups. The following descriptions are very brief and intended to whet your appetite for further learning:

Traditionalists aka Seniors or Veterans (Born before 1945)

- Events of Influence: World War I, the Great Depression, World War II
- Characteristics: hard work, loyalty, sacrifice, thriftiness, working fast to meet deadlines. Expected the workplace to take care of them for life.
- What nurse managers need to know about them: They prefer to have decisions explained, and clearly defined structures. They also have a tendency for black-and-white think-

ing, follow procedures exactly as outlined, and require support and recognition of accomplishments.

Baby Boomers (Born before 1965)

- Events of Influence: Vietnam War, Cold War, assassination of JFK, space exploration, the sexual revolution, drugs, and rock 'n' roll.
- Characteristics: Personal fulfillment, optimism, crusades; buy now, pay later, live to work. Changing jobs frequently looked upon as a sign of "personal instability."
- What nurse managers need to know about them: Most prefer defined structures and clear expectations. flexibility, and recognition. They want to be left alone! They are disillusioned, tired, and have low-to-no trust in the workplace. They want their pay and are on a countdown to their pensions. Some are retired and still on the job. Many live with their adult children who have moved out, come back (sometimes with *their* children), and are affectionately known as Boomerangs. This recent family phenomenon is now creating additional pressures for Seniors and Boomers.

Generation X (Born before 1980)

- Events of Influence: These were the first latchkey kids, who often came home to empty houses. Many are from single parent or both parents working families. The energy crisis and turbulent economic times created instability in the job market, leaving this generation to witness the effects of their parents being laid off as companies downsized. In turn, this generation was left with a strong ethic of self-reliance, disillusionment, and little confidence in the belief (unlike their baby Boomer parents) that the organization in which they worked would not take care of them. When criticized by Boomers as being disloyal, is it any wonder?

- Characteristics: Well-educated, technologically savvy, and independent (they had to be with getting lunches on their own, using microwave ovens, and often looking after younger siblings until a parent arrived home).

- What nurse managers need to know about them: They are goal oriented, money focused, work to live, prefer to work independently, and love project work. They want frequent feedback to determine if their career goals are on track and will change jobs to meet their goals or if they are not treated well. They want rewards, recognition, flexibility, and the ability to use technology.

Generation Y aka Millennials (Born after 1980)

- Events of Influence: Boomers gave them everything, including the latest technology, designer clothes, videogames and tons of praise. They participated in numerous activities as children, were encouraged to express their feelings, and spoke out. They are globally aware thanks to instant and 24-hour media coverage of events such as the Gulf War and ecological disasters.

- Characteristics: They are collaborators, team players, high performers if motivated, and techno wizards. They have a "can-do attitude." They tend not to respond to command-and-control leadership and become easily bored. They also want flexibility, worklife balance, and respond well to change.
- What nurse managers need to know about them: They thrive on challenges and can handle more than one task at a time. They expect a coach, a mentor, a friend, not a "boss." They want respect, honesty, and to work for ethical and environmentally responsible organizations. And by the way, they "just wanna have fun."

WHAT THE GENERATIONS
CAN OFFER EACH OTHER

1. **Silent/Veterans**: This generation "has seen it all." Because many of them valued loyalty and remained with an organization for decades, they bring the perspective of history to the practice setting. While some may regard them as "dinosaurs in the system," they can also be viewed as sources of inspiration because of their character and experience!

2. **Baby Boomers**: Many freely admit they are ready to retire, although the recent economic downturn is causing many to rethink their retirement plans. This generation has been downsized, reengineered, and pummeled with organizational change. Nurse managers must think about the impact of workload and the physical demand being placed on aging Baby Boomers who choose to extend their worklives.

Boomers posses a wealth of knowledge and skills that make them ideal for providing lighter, less demanding, care while serving as mentors and coaches to younger or less experienced staff.

3. **Generation X:** Because they are independent, project oriented, and innovative, they are natural leaders in implementing or facilitating change in the workplace. While many nurse managers are swamped with numerous commitments, Gen Xers are chomping at the bit waiting to be asked to assume a project or take charge of a situation.

4. **Generation Y/Millennials:** These are your "go to techno wizards," who are creative, want to help others to belong and make a difference. Who better to help in the implementation of technology related to patient care?

JUST TELL ME WHAT YOU WANT, WHAT YOU REALLY, REALLY WANT

Most people regardless of their generation want:

- To be treated with dignity and respect.
- To be treated fairly.
- To have opportunities to learn at work and be asked for their opinion.
- To be recognized for jobs well done and told "thank you."
- To have their needs recognized and understood by their nurse manager.
- To receive constructive feedback.
- To be asked for their opinion

GOT GAP?

Strategies for nurse managers in bridging the generational gap:

1. Scan your workplace for the types and numbers in your generational mix.
2. Develop a plan to meet the generational communication needs for your staff by reflecting on the tools you currently use for communicating. Are they effective? Is there room for improvement? Ask each staff member for their input and ideas.
3. Determine how each staff member can best use his or her generation-based "gifts" to contribute to addressing the challenges in the workplace and improving patient care.
4. Be mindful of the underbelly of negative interpersonal dynamics among the generations in your workplace.
5. Create opportunities for conversations about the generations (i.e. staff meetings or nursing in-service). Discuss how generational differences impact relationships between nurses, and patients and among nursing staff.
6. If you want to pair the generations on a project or in providing nursing care, try combining a Senior and Generation Xer or match a Gen Yer with a Boomer. These pairings have more in common than you or they may think.
7. Manage generation bashing when you hear it by stating something like this, "This is not how we talk about our professional colleagues in our workplace."

Fast facts in a nutshell

- How well multigenerations of nurses work together will depend on how well the nurse manager engages staff in creating a respectful workplace, understands what makes each group tick, and inspires staff to believe that together they are better!

CRISIS OR OPPORTUNITY?

The reality for many is that the shifting demographics of a multigenerational staff could lead to both interpersonal crises or incredible opportunities among staff. As a crisis, the situation will invite differing expectations, tension, conflict, hurtful behaviors, and poor quality of care. However, the same situation led and managed by an inspired nurse manager, could create opportunities for generational cross-pollination, coaching and mentoring between the generations, creative initiatives for quality improvement, and fun.

Creating opportunities for mixed generational groups to sit down and talk to each other about what they value about each generation, what behaviors of each generations challenges them, and what strengths each generation brings to the workplace is a healthy way to promote understanding. It also promotes staff learning and professional growth.

**AND THEY ALL LIVED HAPPILY EVER AFTER
THE END**

Fast facts in a nutshell: summary

- When nurse managers require mutual respect, understanding, and acceptance of diversity among their multigenerational staff members, they demonstrate and live the standards inherent in their Codes of Ethics and Standards of Professional Practice.

Chapter 6

"It Was the Best of Times; It Was the Worst of Times. . . ."

Managing and Facilitating Change and Transitions

INTRODUCTION

The ability to facilitate change and manage transitions is a relatively new competency for nurse managers. Formerly left to senior leaders and change management gurus, nurse managers were often left to deal with the impact of change and the fallout from the staff's transition. Nurse managers who understand the potential impact of organizational change on the psychological transitions of their nursing staff and the workplace culture are better able to respond in a proactive and supportive manner.

In this chapter, you will learn:

1. The importance of understanding the human impact of organizational change.

2. How psychological transitions influence staff behaviors in the workplace.
3. Strategies for facilitating change in your practice setting.

THE METAPHORIC TRAIN OF CHANGE IS COMIN' DOWN THE TRACK

To truly understand staff's perception of organizational change, view it within the context of the metaphor of the "train is leaving the station." Here, staff are invited to "hop on," baggage and all, lay down on the tracks, or remain on the platform, which, by the way, is about to be burned! If you can visualize the feelings that accompany this journey, such as fear of the unknown and what will work look like at the end of the journey, then you are well on your way to developing a plan for managing change and transition.

THE RIPPLE EFFECT OF ORGANIZATIONAL CHANGE

The degree of impact of organizational change on staff depends on several factors, including the frequency of change, staff experience with past change, and how well change was managed by leadership. If change is occurring in a remote area of the workplace, other staff may respond with the casual interest of a bystander. If, however, the change is imposed on them, staff members may experience a variety of responses and feelings, including powerlessness, disrespect, and anger that may not be obvious. When these feelings prevail, quality of worklife takes a direct hit and may quickly turn into a workplace dominated by anger, frustration, apathy, low self-esteem, resistance to change, and in-fighting.

At the same time, the work ethic of caring that nurses normally extended to their peers, patients, and clients may assume a narrower focus if their energies are directed exclusively toward patient care and self-preservation. This leaves little room for or interest in supporting their colleagues and organizational change initiatives.

NURSES' ANGER

Nurse managers must recognize the depth of emotions the staff feels about work and nurses' potential for harbouring a deep-seated, often unexpressed, anger. Until recently, women's anger has not been particularly well researched. Thomas, Smucker, and Droppleman (1998) shed light on the fact that **anger develops in women as the result of an accumulation of feelings associated with "hurt, frustration and disillusionment"** (p. 311). They also described the medical impact of nurses' unresolved anger that may lead to conditions such as hypertension, obesity, and migraine headaches. **As nurse manager, it may be more than a passing interest to note the possibility of a connection among organizational change, nurses' anger, the health of nurses, and the quality of worklife.**

KNOW YOUR WORKPLACE CULTURE

As nurse manager, how do you help nurses step back from their frenetic pace and acknowledge their situation, name their feelings, and restore their sense of caring power when the pressures of organizational change are bearing down?

One strategy is **to conduct a cultural assessment of your practice setting** to determine staff readiness to accept change. Once you determine where staff fit on the acceptance scale, you can identify what staff will need to engage in the change process. The following questions may help you identify potential "hot spots" and point you toward some steps to help staff adapt and embrace a new way of being.

1. How content is the staff?
2. How well do staff members work together?
3. Is there a spirit of cooperation, collaboration, and support, or is there conflict, tension, and in-fighting?
4. Are staff members resistant to change because they are fed up, tired, burned out, or do not trust the process?
5. What patterns of resistance might you anticipate?
6. Who are the formal and informal leaders among your staff?
7. What kind of influence do these leaders exert?
8. Which staff members are most likely to support organizational change?
9. What roles can these informal leaders play in positively influencing others?
10. What type of language is reflected in your workplace? Is it upbeat, positive, and professional, or does it reflect negativity, victimization, and resistance? How often do you hear staff refer to "they" and "them"?

SMART MESSENGERS DON'T GET SHOT

'Tis a perilous journey one takes when delivering a message of impending change. But it does not have to be. The following scenario may help you in crafting and delivering a message of change:

> Your practice area is about to be affected by a dramatic organizational change process, with no changes in staff. How do you communicate and prepare staff members for acceptance and engagement and lay the groundwork for change with the least amount of disruption and upheaval? The following ponderables are offered for your consideration.

DON'T TELL: FACILITATE!

When you think about managing change that affects your practice setting, it is important to know that **a more traditional command-and-control style of leading is less effective than facilitating, coaching, mentoring and, yes, counseling** (within your scope of practice).

When organizational change is imposed, nurse managers may have little time to learn expert skills to facilitate the process. They can, however, draw on their principles of therapeutic communication to achieve a running start in helping staff manage a new workplace reality. Facilitating creates an environment in which individuals are helped to name their experiences, engage in dialogue about their situation, and transform their world, according to Freire (1997). How do you find the time to create these opportunities? The real question that requires an answer is not how, but when?

Fast facts in a nutshell

- Facilitating true dialogue creates opportunities for reflection, empathic listening, exchanging ideas, laughter, and professional growth.
- Dialogue opens the door for increased self-awareness and promotes camaraderie.

CRASH COURSE IN FACILITATION 101

Nurses are natural facilitators. Here is a refresher on how you do it—your crash course in facilitation. **Facilitation is a process that requires you to help participants assess their needs, encourage meaningful conversations, develop collaborative interventions, strengthen workplace relationships and create positive outcomes that benefit all!**

1. Consider the following metaphor and visualize your entire staff sitting before you as a patient who is facing surgery and expressing fear, denial, and anger. What nursing diagnoses would you attribute to "your patient"? What would your nursing interventions include? What outcomes would you anticipate? How would you evaluate the outcomes?
2. Developing your plan for facilitation: create opportunities for dialogue (roundtable conversations work great), invite feedback from small groups to share with the larger group, listen for key messages, listen for what is not being said, help staff distil their messages, and facilitate the develop-

ment of an action plan and steps for follow-up. Basically, listen more than you speak; repeat what they said for clarity (for example, "this is what I hear you saying . . . Is that correct?), and write down what they say.

3. For change to be accepted staff will need:

   a. A compelling reason to change. Help nurses answer the question, "Why change?"

   b. Lots of information to support the reasons for change, such as data and stories.

   c. Opportunities to become involved.

   d. Communication, communication, and more communication.

   e. Do not rely solely on memos. Staff could be drowning in them, and someone will with just a hint of indignation will say, "I never saw that!"

   f. Clear expectations. Tell them what you expect from them and yourself. Ask them if your expectations of you are consistent with theirs.

   g. Opportunities to celebrate small and big successes.

   h. Empathy for staff's thoughts and feelings.

This is not intended to be an all-inclusive list, but it will give you a fair of idea about what to look for and include in your staff's journey toward successful implementation. Once you have assessed the workplace culture and your staff's state of readiness for change, you can develop your plan of action that supports changes initiative.

SNAGS, ROADBLOCKS, AND WORKPLACE VARMINTS

We all know the expression: "The best laid plans of mice and men. . . ." Therefore, **expect the best of outcomes in planned change, but don't be surprised if an obstacle rears its ugly head.** Delays happen as well. When these occur, remind yourself that you have a choice in how you view the situation. It can be either a crisis or an opportunity! Sometimes snags are blessings in disguise. Instead of getting your knickers in a twist, step back and ask yourself, "What are the opportunities and possibilities that exist right now at this moment? Think about it then seize the moment!

Remember during the implementation of your plan, be creative, listen well, and be empathetic. Face-to-face meetings are the best venue for communicating with staff. Offer bulleted lists that include "just the fact's M'am" and any other strategies that you can conjure up to grab your multigenerational staff's attention and hold their interest. One more thing, if your sense of humour is dormant, wake it up!

FOLLOW THE LEADER: LEADING CHANGE

If you are tasked with the responsibility for leading a change initiative, know that your greatest challenge will come not from the hard issues related to the design or developmental phases of change management, but rather from the soft or human response. In the end, **successful change management is less about processes and operations and more about managing**

the mindsets of the staff to prepare and fully engage in planned change.

A number of excellent templates can guide you in planning the change management process. John Kotter, Peter Block, William Bridges, and Rick Maurer all offer models and valuable insights into managing change, steps to be taken, guides for conversations, achieving engagement, and managing resistance.

CHANGE CAN BE HARD:
TRANSITIONS CAN BE HARDER

One of the toughest realities for managers and staff to accept is the constancy of change. When change and the ensuing psychological transitions are well managed, nurse managers and their staffs achieve a strategic and patient-care advantage. When you are prepared to expect and manage a variety of reactions from staff, don't neglect your own transitions.

MANAGING CHANGE IS ABOUT MANAGING
AND TRANSFORMING MINDSETS

- In a changing workplace, we are all on a learning curve toward a paradigm shift that will transform how we think about work and how we get the work done.
- We have the power to choose our attitude.
- Attitude is a symptom of a psychological mindset.

- Mindsets include our self-concept, values, self-esteem, and beliefs, as well as how we perceive our world.
- Deal with your mindset first and then the staffs'.

KNOWLEDGE IS POWER

The more we know about the change process and the psychological transitions we go through in response to change, the more prepared we are to prevent and manage unhealthy staff responses, poor quality of care, and deteriorating quality of worklife. As human beings, we are inclined to be creatures of habit. Thus, when change is anticipated or introduced, we react with a broad range of thoughts, feelings, and behaviors, ranging from joy to despair. William Bridges in his book *Managing Transitions: Making the Most of Change,* published in 1991 when there were few books on the subject, was among the first to identify the human response to organizational change. Although many excellent reference books have been written on change management, Bridges offers ponderables for your consideration and a practical framework for helping managers and staff navigate the change process, weather the storms of transitions, see the possibilities, celebrate successes, and prepare for the next round of change.

Fast facts in a nutshell

- According to William Bridges (1991): humans + change = psychological transition
- Transition is a psychological process that individuals go through to manage and adapt to change.
- Change is about attitudes, feelings, and behaviors.

WHEN CHANGE BEGINS, TRANSITIONS FOLLOW

Change is inevitable in today's workplaces, but **change without successful transition initiatives can be doomed to failure.** According to Bridges, every change is accompanied by a psychological response known as the transition process. The rate at which individuals progress through those phases will vary, as will the length of time they spend in each phase. Transition occurs whether change is perceived as "good" or "bad." According to Bridges, the three phases of transitions consist of Endings, the Neutral Zone, and New Beginnings. While some staff will hold onto the past by refusing to move forward, others will progress along the transition continuum toward the next phase, where chaos and confusion are the order of the day as staff members struggle to accommodate the changes they are required to make. Eventually most will embrace new rules, new roles, and new competencies.

The next three chapters create opportunities to enlighten nurse managers about key behaviors typically observed on the transition continuum and how to manage them.

Fast facts in a nutshell: summary

- The more nurse managers know about managing the change process, the more likely staff members are to engage in the change initiative.
- Regard change management as a road trip and a journey to our future. Some roads will be rocky, others will be smooth, and, in some cases, side roads will need to be explored. Some side roads may enrich the journey, while others may cause us to turn back and "course correct."

Chapter 7

It's Over

Managing the End of Old Ways of Being

INTRODUCTION

One of the advantages of good teamwork is the familiarity that team members have with one another. They know whom to call upon when they need help, need a good laugh, want to celebrate their successes, or need a shoulder to cry on. When change is introduced, routines and staff relationships are often disrupted. This chapter outlines common staff responses, explanations, and strategies for helping staff manage what happens when the once familiar is gone.

In this chapter, you will learn:

1. The impact of change when a former way of being must give way to a new.
2. What behaviors to look for when staff is faced with the end of what was once familiar.
3. Tips for helping staff let go of the past.

THE TRAIN HAS LEFT THE STATION: ONE JOURNEY ENDS AND ANOTHER BEGINS

The old way of being is no more! It is over. **Depending on the significance of the impending change, these words can create no response, a mere ripple, or send shock waves through an organization or workplace.** Even though this may be anticipated when changes impact clinical practice or workplace relationships, staff will still react. Some will be excited about the possibilities that change can bring, while others may experience disbelief, betrayal, anger, grief, loss, and/or fear.

BIG MISTAKE

With the announcement of impending organizational change, well-meaning leaders invest a great deal of energy carefully crafting the message in such a way as to get staff "buy-in." They may attempt to "rally the troops" with the familiar battle cry, "People! The train is leaving the station." When staff members hear this, they will probably feel railroaded into accepting the impending change, and feelings of suspicion, anger, resistance, and powerlessness take hold. Resistance is guaranteed.

IT'S NOT WHAT YOU HEAR, IT'S WHAT YOU DON'T HEAR THAT COUNTS

As you consider communication about change, keep in mind that verbal communication comprises only 7% of an interaction. Therefore, **staff member's verbal responses of support to messages about change may mask underlying and unexpressed feelings.** During this time, nurse managers are well advised to listen carefully to what the staff is not saying, observe nonverbal actions, and be open to a bailiwick of fascinating reactions.

FASCINATING COMMENTS YOU MAY HEAR

A. "But it ain't broke, why fix it?"
When staff is overheard making the remark, "it ain't broke," it is a clear signal of a communication gap between the intent of the message and what is perceived. It may also reflect blame that staff members are inclined to assign when they do not see the benefit of impending change. Some nurse managers will mistakenly try to convince staff that their perceptions are wrong when they hear these comments.

B. Another "Flavor of the Month"
Depending on the amount and frequency of change staff has experienced, don't be surprised if nurses reflect a high level of cynicism when told about the latest change. They may refer to the pronouncement as a "flavor-of-the-month" initiative. This usually indicates that the staff does not see the value of the proposed change and has little faith in a successful outcome. This remark also speaks to a lack of trust in leadership. What staff may really be saying is, "I do not see the need for this change, I don't have enough information, I don't understand, or I don't trust you."

C. "I can't believe this? Where is this coming from?"
This comment can reflect staff's level of awareness about what is happening in the organization, the timing of the message, or how the message is delivered.

D. "Been there, done that, bought the tee shirt."
While a comment like this seems resistant and dismissive, it actually serves as a cue that the information received may not be what was intended or that this most recent change is no change at all in the minds of some. Some staff members have been around long enough to believe that they've "seen and done it all." The danger lies in the potential of this comment to influence others in a negative way. How much this remark impacts the peer group depends on how much power the individual who makes this remark has.

THINGS YOU MAY SEE

A. Breaking up is hard to do.
Many staff members will state that their peer group at work is like their second family. When staff groups are forced to separate because of organizational change, the loss can be so profound that the grief and anger can last for years.

Some nurses have more to lose than others when the group is disbanded. Depending on the nature of their workplace relationships, some individuals will lose real or perceived power and/or status. This can be threatening to the group, particularly if the change means they will lose their "informal leader." When the sense of loss at work is this severe, the potential for individual and group depression is very real. Change cannot successfully be absorbed until the underlying issues related to grief and loss are dealt with in a compassionate manner.

B. When the nurse manager is downsized or redeployed.
When staff loses a beloved nurse manager, the sense of loss is profound. Feelings of anger and grief run very deep and may persist for years if not acknowledged, named, and dealt with appropriately. Chronically negative workplace relationships can result in a mindset that the "new" manager will never fill the void. Successive nurse managers may face huge resistance and staff rejection. Dealing with this type of anger and loss will require patience, understanding, skilful handling, and refocusing the staff's attention on the provision of excellent care.

C. Fear of the unknown.
Many staff members have a high need for order and predictability. Not knowing what lies ahead can induce mild to severe anxiety and behaviors that reflect any number of symptoms, including decreased productivity, complaining, irritability, and increasing use of sick time. Fear of making a "career limiting move" may cause some individuals to become nonparticipative, go through the motions, or mentally "shut down."

D. Real and perceived loss.
It is safe to assume that there may be numerous real and perceived losses experienced when something is over. Loss can be associated with the threat of or actual job loss, personal or professional status (because of role or job change), peer group power dynamics, giving up the familiar, and the introduction of new equipment or processes.

Fast facts in a nutshell

- When a way of being is over, staff may struggle with losing or changing familiar patterns, issues of power and control, relationships, and ways of thinking.
- Whatever staff members perceive is their reality. The language staff uses to express these perceptions should never be dismissed lightly. It is the nurse managers job to help staff express and name what lies beneath their seemingly off-handed comments.

THREE STATEMENTS YOU SHOULD NEVER UTTER WHEN SOMETHING ENDS

Guaranteed, you will shake staff's sense of trust in you if you say any one of the following:

1. **You**: "Trust me; this change will be a good thing."
   Staff's unspoken response: "No we won't trust you, you are 'management's messenger,' you report to senior management, and they have the power to fire you and us."
2. **You**: "We need your buy-in."
   Staff's unspoken response, "I am not so sure I want to 'buy' anything right now. You sound like a used car salesman and who trusts them?"
3. **You**: "I can't talk about that right now."
   Staff's unspoken response: "Hmmm. There must be something 'they' are holding back. They are probably going to

fire us all or close the service. I better start looking for another job!" You can never really trust management!"

TIPS FOR LETTING GO

1. Reflect on your position within the context of endings. Do you support the proposed changes? How prepared are you to deal with the tough emotional issues of staff? How do you go through the motions of supporting change when you do not agree with the strategy? How will that influence staff? What do you need to do to manage your personal acceptance of the proposed changes? What resources do you need to call on to support you and your staff as you move forward?
2. Tell the truth.
3. Acknowledge and manage your own and your staff's anger and grief associated with loss.
4. Help staff to reflect on and let go of the past. What was good about the old way of being? What needed improvement? Explore how this change might be an improvement.
5. Manage resistance.
6. Create an Open Door policy so that staff members can drop in to express their feelings. When they do, help them determine what steps are necessary for them to move forward.
7. Reinforce reality by giving staff information, data, costs, and other details. If the change is about the "bottom line," show staff your budget printouts.
8. Ask the question, "Why change?," and then ask staff members to answer it.

9. Provide staff with a brief bulleted list of the issues and the overall organizational plan (no more than six points on a page) for moving forward.

10. Remind staff that when change is inevitable; it will happen whether or not they approve.

11. Remind them also that accepting change is uncomfortable for most of us. It is okay to feel that way for a while, but they will have to move on sooner rather than later.

12. Commit to communicate, communicate, and communicate (tell; write; tell again).

13. Make yourself available to answer questions. Discourage the use of the grapevine and encourage them to come to you or check things out themselves.

14. If you don't know the answer to a question, tell them so and that you will find out and get back to them as soon as possible.

15. If change is going to alter your unit culture by introducing more staff or moving staff to other areas, gather the staff together before the change occurs and discuss the following:
    - What are the accomplishments we most are most proud of as a unit?
    - What improvements do we feel need to happen to improve our practice or quality of service?
    - How will the impending changes improve our service?
    - What obstacles might we face during this improvement?
    - What plans can we make to celebrate our past?

16. Remember: It is not what you say; it's what you do. Staff will be watching you very closely to see if your actions match your words. (How upbeat are you about these

changes? Do your words reflect support for the organization's direction? If you are angry about change, is it showing?)

Suggestions for celebrating what once was: Create a scrapbook or a photo album of past events or create a social event to celebrate the past and welcome the future.

Fast facts in a nutshell: summary

- Successful transition from a former way of being is mostly about managing the mindsets of staff members. The "soft" issues frequently associated with change are fear, letting go, grief and loss, celebrating and honoring the past, and paving the way to the new normal of chaos and confusion, as staff journeys toward a new or different way of being and working.

Chapter 8

Now What?

Managing Chaos and Confusion

INTRODUCTION

Once change has been introduced to your staff as inevitable, the main task of you and the staff is to "make it work." Meet your new best friends: Chaos and Confusion! This chapter describes some of the antics that staff members may craft in response to their emerging new reality and offers insights and tips for managing their innovative and occasionally challenging behavior.

In this chapter, you will learn:

1. How chaos and confusion impacts individuals as they move toward a new way of being.
2. Tips for managing chaos and confusion.

THE PERILOUS JOURNEY OF CHAOS AND CONFUSION ON THE ROCKY MOUNTAIN RAILROAD!

If you have ever taken Disneyland's Rocky Mountain Railroad ride you have been initiated into the world of surprises, obstacles, and exhilaration. This is what follows the introduction of planned change! The metaphoric train of change has left the station loaded with a mix of anxious, excited, and a few reluctant passengers. They are embarking on a journey to somewhere, but they are unsure about what the destination will look like. Little do they know that along the way they may be faced with perils of frightening proportions. They know that they cannot turn back, and the trip will get worse before it gets better!

Remember the boulders that threatened to crush you on the ride, the steep slow climb up the mountain, and the train's rapid and shaky descent, which was followed by crossing the ravine on the rickety bridge before finally reaching the station? As they jumped off the train, most passengers were smiling and excited. A few, however, seemed dazed and shaken. In a few instances, a small number of brave passengers quickly ran to catch the next train for another exciting ride! This pretty much sums up the journey of transition from the old to new way of being.

As the metaphoric conductor, your job is to make the passengers as comfortable as possible in the journey ahead. In other words to support staff as they prepare for things to get messy, uncomfortable, and at times downright ugly! Knowing that this phase can be rough gives you a heads up on how to manage the obstacles you may face.

THINGS YOU MAY HEAR ALONG THE JOURNEY OF CHAOS AND CONFUSION

A. "H-E-L-L-L-P!

B. "Just tell us what to do!"
In the "muck and the mire" of chaos and confusion frustration can be the norm and feelings of powerlessness playing out in a number of ways. In merging staff groups, territorial battles and power struggles can develop as individuals focus their energy on the tasks of nursing practice and attempt to determine whose way is better.

C. "Show me the policy!"
When organizations merge, multiple policy and procedure manuals are supposed to merge as well, but this rarely happens fast enough. In the meantime, when nurses are challenged by a practice issue and go looking for the correct policy or procedure to follow, they may find several or none. When this happens, staff can feel confused, anxious, and frustrated.

D. "That's not my job! If you make me do it, I'll grieve!"
This "line-in-the-sand" response is an indicator of the distress staff members feel as they move through this tumultuous period causing them to seek clarity and direction so they can forge new pathways. Even though solid plans and implementation strategies may be in place, there are no sure-fire rules for managing successful change. There are only guidelines.

E. "I'm tired of all this change. I just want to nurse to my patients!"
Staff members are more inclined to draw into themselves during this phase. They become "me" focused and have little energy to spread around. They are in survival mode, and their morale may plummet. They feel patients are being cheated with respect to quality of care and feel guilty about it, but they are not motivated enough to change.

F. "I don't like this. I wanna' go back to the good ol' days."
Wanting to return to the familiar is natural. What is not natural is to sabotage progress or be angry enough to negate change efforts.

THINGS YOU MAY SEE

A. Polarized staff
If change requires you to bring two or more distinct staff groups together, expect that their natural inclination will be to band together in their groups of origin. Turf wars, competition about which is the better group of nurses, and nasty comments are all expressions of staff struggles with adapting to a new way of being. Teamwork can suddenly go the way of the dodo bird!

B. Increased use of sick time
Mixed emotions, accommodating different practices, and mental and physical exhaustion can cause staff to more readily call in sick and be less likely to "go the extra mile."

C. Following the informal leader

According to Bridges, this is when people struggle with ambiguity, look for answers that may not be there, and readily attach themselves to someone who is authoritative, seems to know what they are doing, and appears competent and confident (p. 39). This is fine, as long as this "new-found" and informal leader is positive, proactive, and aligned with the direction of the organization. If this person is negative, reactive, and undermining your leadership, you may be facing a potential power struggle.

Fast facts in a nutshell

- Staff members are more willing to embrace change when they see how it will improve practice or patient/client care.
- There are always a few staff who can only focus on themselves. They try to maintain the status quo and just wait for a "return to the way things were."

THE GOOD NEWS

When staff recognizes that in-fighting and power struggles are a bad use of good energy and decide to work together for the good of the patient, the seeds are sown for collaboration and creativity in the newly defined workplace. The train is headed for solid ground.

Fast facts in a nutshell

- Expect chaos and confusion in the time between what was and what will be.
- During the phase of chaos and confusion, staff members may look for answers when there are none.
- Things will get better.

MANAGING CHAOS, CONFUSION, AND ANYTHING ELSE THROWN YOUR WAY

1. Reinforce reality by clearly communicating the following messages to staff members:
   - Yes, this is difficult but we have to move forward.
   - Determine whether you are thriving or merely surviving.
   - Ask staff if they are merely surviving the journey or are thriving?
   - Ask them what surviving looks like, and ask them what thriving looks like.
   - Recommend that they choose to thrive!
   - Have a conversation about what actions and behaviors support thriving.
   - Tell staff members that they have the power to choose their attitude on this journey.
   - Remind staff that when organizational change occurs, some decisions are negotiable, and some are not. Individuals may have input into how something is done, but they may not have the authority to determine

whether something will be done. Make sure staff understands which is which!

2. Educate staff about transitions.

3. Set both short- and long-term goals for implementation of initiatives.

4. Look for opportunities to identify emerging leaders and provide opportunities for the development of individuals in temporary leadership roles.

5. Clarify what policies and procedures must be followed at this time. Explain that they are never a substitute for critical thinking and professional practice.

6. Check your generation mix: Have you got a Gen Xer leading an initiative or with a project team? Did you pair your Gen Yers with some Boomers?

7. Continue regular verbal and written progress reports and acknowledge successes.

8. Be available and visible to help individuals maintain their focus on implementing change, while never losing sight of their patients.

9. When staff members seems stuck or the Go Forward plan gets derailed, offer a time out to review why things are off track and invite their input with, "Let's figure out how we can get back on track."

10. In collaboration with staff, create activities and celebrations that promote connections and collegiality.

11. Facilitate discussions about what individuals have in common—the values they share and their beliefs about nursing practice.

12. Reinforce that there are no mistakes; there are only opportunities to learn as you make your way through this change.

13. Continue with regular meetings for communication updates.
14. Conduct a self-check-in about how you are feeling. Are you taking care of yourself?

NEWS FLASH! YOU ARE NOT PERFECT, YOU ARE ONLY HUMAN

Sometimes your plate can be too full as you try to be all things to all people. You feel that if anyone asks you to do one more thing, you just might explode. If you fear that this is the case, you may have to put on the emergency brakes, take stock of what you have onboard, shift your cargo, or make some priority decisions about what can be temporarily left behind.

Unless you strongly believe that you might be making a career limiting move, discuss this situation (using a written plan) with the person to whom you report using the following format:

1. Identify the issue of overload and give examples.
2. State why it is important to address this issue
3. Describe what the benefits would be if you "course correct."
4. Make some recommendations about steps you would like to take.
5. Identify anticipated outcomes.
6. Identify timelines for completion or resolution of the issue.
7. Tell your boss that you will give them regular updates on your progress.
8. Once your plan is approved, share it with staff.

> ## Fast facts in a nutshell
>
> - When you take on too much and try to please everyone, you end up paying a high price. The inability to recognize when you are experiencing work overload can lead to the breakdown of change processes, workplace relationships, and you!
> - Just say, "No!" Although it may seem difficult to say, it is after all only a one syllable word!

ARRIVING AT YOUR NEW DESTINATION

As you and the staff get closer to your destination, take pride in your progress, how well you survived the journey, and the realization that as a group, you just might be better now than you were before. You will experience more positive behavior among most of the staff as you settle in and become comfortable with your new way of being. There may be a few staff who have not engaged, and they are the focus of future discussion.

The bottom line is that once you've mastered the chaos and confusion and completed the journey, the worst is over until the next set of changes comes knocking at your door.

Fast facts in a nutshell: summary

- When the train of organizational change traverses the perilous terrain of chaos and confusion, it eventually reaches the destination of a new way of being. When that happens, pat yourselves on the back, celebrate the journey, and prepare for absorbing the new ways of being, new collaborative relationships, and improved outcomes in service delivery. What's not to like?

Chapter 9

From Isolation to Collaboration

Managing a New Way of Being

INTRODUCTION

Once you have managed the predictable chaos and confusion over the introduction of something or someone new, you can expect a period of respite where calm and serenity prevail. Be assured that it will only last until the next round of changes. This chapter celebrates movement away from egocentricity and chaos toward alignment, collaboration, and overall acceptance of a new way of being.

In this chapter, you will learn:

1. The signs that change is beginning to embed.
2. Strategies for managing the beginning of a new way of being.

A NEW WAY OF BEING IS JUST ON THE HORIZON

Managing your own and staff transitions is one of the most difficult challenges facing nurse managers. After this phase is completed, do not be fooled into thinking that implementation and embedding of the changes "is the easy part." Do not compare it to the challenges you faced in ending the old ways of being and helping individuals work through the confusion that occurs when two systems, ideologies, or practices collide. Being tuned into the psychological impact of changes at work provides you and your staff with opportunities for new learning, professional growth, and the chance to make meaningful change.

With chaos and confusion diminishing and territorial battles won and lost, staff members begin to accept the inevitable—that a new way of being is just around the corner. Whole-scale acceptance by and engagement of all staff is unlikely and will vary among staff in the early stages of the new beginning. When the uptake is slow or becomes temporarily derailed, the cynics will shout with glee, "I told you this wouldn't work!" More likely, they will develop a smugness rivaled only by the Mona Lisa.

Depending on the mindset of the naysayers and resistors, the implementation and embedding phase may be at risk for complete failure, as the potential for a renewed power struggle lurks on the sidelines.

THE PROBLEM WITH IMPLEMENTING
PLANNED CHANGE

Planned change usually has a strategic planning committee hovering in the background, much like family members anticipating the birth of a first child. To assist in the delivery is an appointed steering committee, whose job is to manage and support the process according to meticulously drafted protocols and tight time lines. The committee's accountability is evidenced in monitoring the course of actions and making "course corrections" to ensure the "deliverable" arrives on schedule. **However, although the implementation plan and schedule may work in theory, the progression of people along the implementation continuum is far less predictable.** Despite "the best laid plans of mice and men," plans can go awry. As nurse managers attempt to manage the people aspect of embedding organizational change, take comfort in the words of Warren Bennis, who said, "Managing people is like herding cats."

Because nurse managers know their staffs best, they must be aware of and anticipate obstacles that may get in the way of launching a new beginning. It is especially important for managers to be there, remain visible, and be open to feedback from staff.

Fast facts in a nutshell

- Accepting the inevitable fact that plans will run amok, timelines will become moving targets, and people won't do what they are supposed to do for a variety of reasons better prepares you to manage the beginning of new way of being.

- Managing your own response as you lead your staff during this phase will require you to call upon a number of competencies that include flexibility, patience, resurrecting your sense of humor, and maintaining a presence of living in the moment.

WILL THE PLANNED CHANGE STICK?

That depends. **Do not be surprised if while the change initiative is still in its infancy, some staff members will revert to old habits** and ways of doing something. For example, if you are introducing an automated system, individuals may secretly use their tried and true, handwritten manual system! This behavior may signal any number of things, including resistance, testing the system for permanency, or testing you. In a system where staff members are bombarded by what they perceive as "flavor-of-the-month" changes, it makes sense for them to test whether or not this change is "for real."

WHAT YOU MAY EXPERIENCE AS YOU AND YOUR STAFF ENGAGE IN A NEW WAY OF BEING

- The focus of staff energy and caring belongs on the patient or client.
- Staff appears more connected to one another.

- Relationships become collaborative rather than territorial.
- The sound of appropriate laughter in your workplace or cafeteria becomes music to your ears.
- Mixed emotions of excitement and anticipatory anxiety may emerge during the launch phase and embedding of changes. Note to self: This is normal.
- The staff members who play a part in developing and implementing the "new way of being" develop a greater sense of ownership and pride in the process and outcomes.
- The leadership potential of staff becomes evident
- Staff members who participate on steering committees with others from across the organization begin to expand their workplace horizons by grasping the "big picture" and interconnectedness of the organization.
- The potential for individuals to become ambassadors of change is greater when they see the value of progress as it relates to their practice and quality of care processes.
- Committed and engaged staff leaders become role models for their peers and may inspire others to become involved in future initiatives
- When staff is encouraged and supported in moving though transitions there is a greater likelihood for personal and professional transformation.

A REFLECTION FOR YOU

"Yesterday is history; tomorrow is a mystery; today is all we have" (unknown source). Throughout the change process, this statement can provide a measure of comfort for you and the staff as you engage in change and move toward a new way of being. By focusing on the present, you ground yourself in the here and now. This helps staff to do the same. In other words, **despite the periodic insanity that can develop during transitions, the one constant is the need for patients and clients to receive excellent care.** Focusing on the present serves to remind you, staff, and the occasional organizational leader of your individual and collective primary responsibility.

TIPS FOR MANAGING STAFF AS THEY EMBARK AND ENGAGE IN A NEW WAY OF BEING

1. Teach and reinforce the principles of managing change, emphasizing that things may not be perfect yet, that everyone is embarking on a new learning curve, and that they may have to be willing to take a leap of faith. Ask them to be patient as you tread boldly where few have gone before!
2. Assess staff members' level of engagement in their new way of being by inviting discussion that highlights improvements in care and the potential for nursing research that will further develop their professional practice.
3. Create opportunities for feedback on what is working well, why is it working well, and what could be done better?
4. Review where everyone was in the good ol' days, and how far we've come. Note achievements and challenges.
5. Initiate a mentoring program.
6. Maintain visibility. Just seeing you present in the workplace can quell feelings of uncertainty and anxiety.
7. Create opportunities for on-going feedback.
8. Continue to talk about and inform staff about the future as you see it—the challenges that you face as manager;

the challenges that you all face as staff, and the challenges that face the organization.

9. Communicate to staff that despite uncertainties, staff members must continue to respect and value one another and work collaboratively. You will to the best of your abilities be available to support their continuing transition.

10. Help staff to celebrate their successes.

11. Remember to say thank you for specific staff achievements and, if you can, handwrite thank-you notes.

12. Hop on the leadership bandwagon! When staff demonstrate effective leadership during the implementation, take note and look for other opportunities for individuals to further develop their new-found skills

13. Keep your eyes open for lingering resistance and/or negative attitudes, and manage them!

14. Continue to monitor the quality of patient/client care.

15. Tell nurses that this is probably not the last they will see and experience of organizational change.

Helping staff navigate transitions is one of the most important competencies for nurse managers to possess in today's changing workplaces. Equally important is being able to manage their own transitions when they are "caught between a rock and a hard place," as they struggle to balance the demands of staff and those of the organization. Leading change requires nurse managers to be self-aware, flexible, risk takers, innovators, and creative. As such, they model the new competencies for a changing world and how to thrive in a changing workplace.

Fast facts in a nutshell: summary

- No one person has all the answers for solving today's complex workplace challenges.
- There is no template for how we proceed toward a new way of being. We've never been here before.
- Since we've never been here before, the only way forward is to work together and do what needs to be done to make the necessary changes happen.

Part III

Staff Gone Wild?
Managing Your Cast of Characters

Chapter 10

Got Resistance?

Expect It! Welcome It! Manage It

INTRODUCTION

Welcome to the murky, energy-zapping world of resistance with its cast of shady characters. How do you recognize and manage overt and covert forms of resistance? This chapter outlines what to look for and how to handle behaviours that can spell trouble if ignored.

In this chapter, you will learn:

1. Resistance is an expected part of change that creates crises and opportunities.
2. The 20/60/20 Rule of Resistance.
3. Basic principles and strategies for removing the masks of resistance.

RESISTANCE IS A NATURAL PARTNER OF CHANGE

Change is inevitable, and so is resistance to it. People resist for any number of reasons, and nurse managers need to recognize it, understand the reasons, and then manage the behaviors. Unchecked resistance can negatively impact staff relationships, affect the quality of worklife and patient care, and jeopardize the success of a change initiative. Among the reasons for resistance are:

1. Fear of the unknown.
2. Perceived threat to the status quo.
3. Perceived threat to image or professional identity.
4. Potential threat to a personal and /or power base.
5. Fear of not being able to do the work that may be required (fear of failure).
6. Fear of being exposed as incompetent.
7. Intentional malfeasance!

In his book, *Beyond the Wall of Resistance (1996),* Rick Maurer, a highly regarded expert in the field of organizational change and resistance, defines resistance as "a force that slows or stops movement" (p. 23). Engaging in or resisting change involves an investment of energy, which for many is a precious commodity and depleted personal resource. Fortunately, the energy required to resist change also has the potential to convert to energy that supports change. Nurse managers are catalysts for that conversion.

KNOW YOUR RESISTANCE HOT SPOTS

Many managers believe that negative comments are "bad" and staff silence and lack of complaining or feedback is "good." While both may be true, so is the opposite. Resistance wears many masks. Overt resistance generally includes what you see and hear, such as verbal protests, endless questions, sarcasm, and excuse making. Resistance becomes especially problematic when it becomes covert. Your nurse manager antenna will tell you that "something is up even though things look fine." You may also hear staff rumblings but you can never pin down the source. Examples of destructive, resistant behaviors include sabotage, such as not showing up for meetings, incomplete tasks related to the change initiative, and deliberate attacks on persons, processes, and equipment. Individuals and groups can demonstrate endless creative capacities to resist change.

Underlying both overt and covert resistance on its deepest level is usually an issue of power and control—personal, group, organizational, or all three. **Dealing with matters of resistance is never optional.** If you are aware that it exists, ignoring it will only give it strength. When nurse managers are informed and mindful of the power dynamics of resistant behavior, they acquire a distinct advantage for facilitating change.

THE 20/60/20 RULE OF RESISTANCE

This simple 20/60/20 Rule of Resistance provides an unscientific yet useful guide for determining the extent of resistance that may be present among your staff. Knowing these approximate percentages and turning on your nurse manager radar will enable you to greet resistance and manage it before it gets out of hand.

The 20% Who Love Change

These individuals thrive in a changing workplace. They are your Champions for Change, your Cheerleaders, and quiet Supporters. They put actions behind their words and do what needs to be done. They are not possessed! Because of their support, however, they can be vulnerable to or held suspect by their peers as "sucking up to the boss!"

The 60% Who Wait and See

When the subject of change is introduced, approximately 60% will sit politely, listen, and appear interested. What happens inside their heads is another matter. This 60% is probably thinking, "How is this change going to mess up my life?" They are neither supporting nor resisting. They quickly move into a "wait-and-see" mode. They need more time to see and believe why change is necessary and may reserve endorsement or engagement until they are convinced. The good news is that in the end this 60% will merge with the keen bean 20% in accepting the proposed change. This 80% now represents a critical mass that is ready to move forward. What about the remaining 20%?

The 20% Who Take 80% of Your Time

Resistance within this group is particularly complex and difficult to manage because the behavior is generally covert in nature. The masks can be anything from smiley faces to Freddy from *Nightmare on Elm Street*. Resistance can sound like support, as for example, in "That seems like a very good plan; you can count on me for support." Don't count on it! Some who say, "That will never work!" may not be resistors. In fact, they may change to supporters. When resistance occurs behind your back, it can turn nasty and has the potential to cause extensive damage to your change management efforts and workplace relationships.

BEWARE THE WORKPLACE SABOTEUR

These most challenging resistors are the (thankfully) rare few who openly "trash" the proposed change, you, the workplace, and the organization. They have no intention of ever supporting the change and make it their mission to ensure that "it" will never happen. These people are not happy campers and will make sure no one else is either. They are especially adept in recruiting physicians to join their fight. These individuals are not poor misguided souls; they are professional saboteurs who will challenge you to your greatest power struggle. They typically possess informal power within the staff, can undermine your authority, and are very difficult to catch in the act.

Permanent night shift can be a hotbed for propagating resistance and recruiting members for "the movement." If you have someone like this on staff, you may not know it. Once you get wind that this situation exists, it must be dealt with. The longer this behavior is allowed to continue the greater the damage—and some of it will be irreparable and, in the end, cause staff to leave.

MANAGING RESISTANCE

So how do you deal with resistance? Watch for it, attempt to understand it, and fearlessly nip it in the bud! The following scenario describes a typical mild-to-moderate expression of resistance from staff.

The stage is set. You are about to deliver an elegant soliloquy on impending change. All players are assembled, and you begin. As you look about the audience, you notice that some have suddenly discovered that their shoes are absolutely fascinating, others are gazing out the window, and one or two valiantly struggle to keep their eyes open while stifling a yawn that threatens to explode their lungs. Bravo! Your message delivery was Tony Award worthy. Feeling confident and comfortable that you communicated the right message to the right people at the right time, you ask if there are any questions. The pause seems as interminable as Simon and Garfunkel's "The Sound of Silence" plays in your head. Finally, some brave soul comments, "Sounds like a good idea to me." Music to your ears! Then a voice from the back mutters, "Been there; done that, bought the tee-shirt," followed by a series of bobblehead nods from those sitting closest to the voice of resistance. You are startled into your own awkward silence.

You are face to face with the masked presence of resistance. **Resistance is not your enemy. In fact, it can be a healthy ally in the process of facilitating change and staff engagement.** The trick is to know the difference and to know that resistance at all levels can be managed.

DON'T BACK DOWN

Organizational change when not managed well can be a catalyst for arousing nurses' anger and a host of other negative responses. **Unresolved and mismanaged anger among nursing staff can lead to resistance toward change, poor quality of care, and disruption in quality of worklife.** As nurse manager, it is vitally important to address staff anger. But many nurse managers are uncomfortable facing this challenge. Here is one reassuring thought. Although snarky comments may sound inappropriate, the fact that they are spoken in front of you may signal that staff members feels safe enough to express themselves in your presence. On the other hand, they may be testing you to see how you will react. **When you hear cynicism, negativity, and nasty asides, always assume that there is more behind those words.** It is your job to find out what lies below! If you ignore this behavior:

1. It will not go away. It will probably get worse and take on a life of its own.
2. It will feed and reinforce staff perception that "management doesn't care" or "they never listen to us anyway."
3. It can create an "us" and "them" situation.

How you respond will determine if the mask comes off and stays off. You can shut down communication with a response such as, "I'm just following orders." (Add drama by throwing your hands in the air!) This is guaranteed to leave staff feeling unsupported, angrier, or more frustrated. Or, you can welcome the remark and open a door to an opportunity for exploring, learning, and mutual growth. When you are *seen* to be comfortable with managing resistance, you inspire confidence and the feeling that "we're in this together."

Fast facts in a nutshell

- Resistance creates opportunities for conversations and personal growth.
- Facilitating meaningful conversations in the presence of resistance is like peeling an onion. Be prepared for multilayers and occasional tears, but the end is worth it.

HANDLING CYNICS, NAYSAYERS, AND DILBERTS

The following dialogue suggests one way to respond to a comment such as, "Here we go again, another flavor-of-the-month initiative!" You can either respond immediately or take some time to think about what you need to say. Sometimes it is helpful to ask individuals to hold their comments until after the presentation, when there will be opportunities for feedback. Or, you can stop your presentation and respond to questions and comments. Each staff and situation is different, and you will have to determine what works best for you.

Take a breath. Acknowledge the person, and say, "What you have to say is important to me. I am hearing that you believe this proposed change is not new and that you don't seem happy with how things went before. I would like to hear more about your experience." Continue using your Communication 101 skills. When you interact with staff in this manner, you are modeling effective relationship principles and competencies. The following describes the potential benefits from this type of healthy conversation:

1. **Demonstrates support for staff**: It tells staff members you are listening, willing to take time to hear what they say, and validates their presence at the meeting.
2. **Demonstrates that you can handle criticism**: It tells staff that it is safe for individuals to express themselves.
3. **Engages staff in meaningful dialogue**: Asking open-ended questions invites two-way conversation.
4. **Builds trust**: At a time when cynicism is rampant and trust in leaders and their decisions can be very low, this approach can restore trust.
5. **Helps you determine the level of resistance among staff**: Sarcastic, cynical, and abrasive remarks are the "tip of the iceberg." Pay attention to body language. Behaviors such as folded arms, crossed legs and eyes rolling backward may be cues that these individuals are disengaging and require follow-up.
6. **Creates an opportunity for you to assess the quality of your communication**: It is important to reflect on the quality of your message, including its delivery, your body

language, staff response, and its impact as staff leave the meeting.

7. **Demonstrates empathy**: When you convey empathy to staff, you reinforce the necessity for nurses to extend empathy to one another.

8. **Creates opportunities to listen for what is not being said**: Only 7% of communication is verbal. What is the message beneath the words? It is your job to find out.

9. **Helps staff name their feelings**: Nurses often struggle with naming what they are *feeling*.

10. **Helps staff learn how to manage feelings**: Conversations about resources to help them manage stress are helpful even though they may be reluctant to admit that they need it.

11. **Facilitates dialogue about what nurses are doing well, what they are proud of, and what they can do better.** Staff can easily get bogged down in the muck and the mire of change. You must create the momentum to keep nurses moving forward. Try saying something like, "That was then, this is now, and the decisions have been made. Our challenge is to make this happen."

12. **Clarifies information about decision making: what is negotiable, and what is not.** Explaining their role in decision making helps staff members understand where their input is welcome. This minimizes their frustration when they voice opinions and receive little or no reaction.

Fast facts in a nutshell: summary

- Listening and responding to what is not being said is a powerful tool of self-discovery for you and your staff.
- When all else fails: If you can't change the people; change the people!

Chapter 11

Got Attitude?

Managing the Good, the Bad, and the Downright Ugly!

INTRODUCTION

An interesting fact of worklife is that many staff members believe that their attitude is the fault of someone or something outside themselves. As a nurse manager, one of your greatest challenges is to manage attitude in the workplace. This chapter will introduce the concept of attitude, the power it can have on the quality of worklife and workplace relationships, and tips for influencing positive change.

In this chapter, you will learn:

1. The impact of attitude in the workplace.
2. The 35/55/10 Attitude Scale: The Good, the Bad, and the Downright Ugly!
3. Basic strategies for managing attitude

WORKPLACE ATTITUDE: GOT SOME?

Attitude in today's workers is pandemic and is best summed up by Antonio, a character from the popular 1990s sitcom *Wings,* who said, "Gaze fondly upon today for tomorrow is bound to suck worse!" Negative attitudes may be a biproduct of change in the workplace and reflect what is really happening at a deeper level with respect to staff feelings, perceptions, and behaviors. **Most often, attitude emanates from feelings of low self-esteem, vulnerability, powerlessness, low trust, a sense of betrayal, disrespect, and mismanagement.**

Attitude is a choice. Regardless of our circumstances at work **each of us has the power to choose our attitude.** The only time we are not held responsible for our attitude is if we are psychotic—and there are medications to treat that! Thriving in a changing workplace largely depends on the attitude staff chooses in response to what is going on in each individual's internal and external environment.

THE GOOD, THE OKAY, AND THE DOWNRIGHT UGLY ATTITUDE SCALE

Change comes with a staff attitude menu that includes: the Good-to-Great, the Okays and So-Sos, and the Downright Ugly. The percentage breakdown on the Attitude Scale is 35/55/10. Although unscientific, it is a good gauge for measuring potential staff attitudes! The numbers reinforce the fact that most of your staff, when led by excellence, will eventually manage whatever changes come their way. But a few never will, and they may give you more than one sleepless night.

The 35% Good-to-Great Attitudes

Part-time nurses seem to be the happiest of all. They readily admit that they can, "Come to work, do my job, and at the end of my shift leave the politics behind, and feel good about what I've accomplished." Many other nurses actively avoid getting involved in "the gossip and back-biting" and focus on patient care. They are very adept at managing peer relationships by "getting along with everyone." When they find themselves in uncomfortable situations (i.e., gossip, bullying, or compromised practice) they will do the right thing. These nurses are your role models for demonstrating healthy workplace relationships and meeting their practice Standards. Your recognition and support is vital to keeping them motivated and engaged in their practice. Be mindful of the optics of recognizing these staff, as those who are negative may perceive your behavior as favoritism. They can then target the individual(s) as "teacher's pet(s)" and make work-life difficult for the nurses who are just "trying to do their jobs."

The 55% Okay-to-So-So Attitudes

When change initiatives are ramping up, the pace is frantic, or staffing is tight, the majority of staff seems to be in survival mode. There may be evidence that application of the professional Standards of Practice is weakening. Professional nursing care is at risk of becoming task focused and routine oriented. Patient/client-centered care, continuity of care, and nursing care plans may also become casualties.

At a time like this, nurses may become vulnerable to the negative attitudes of a few but powerful staff. When negativity abounds, most staff "go with the flow" to avoid trouble or to avoid causing problems. This situation can lead to their unwitting participation in creating toxic workplaces. For example, when there is bullying in the workplace, individuals who are not directly involved know what is happening but say nothing for fear of "rocking the boat" or risking the wrath of the bully. In adopting this stance, they become bystanders and accomplices in the bullying process.

When nurses experience negative attitudes and behaviors among their colleagues, they often feel the need to do or say something. However, they are reluctant for fear of disrupting the relationships on which they regularly depend. Others feel unsure about what to say or how to handle negative and toxic situations. While staff may be vulnerable to negative influences at this time, they are equally open to positive ones. This is particularly true when nurse mangers deal with unacceptable behavior and create opportunities for staff to talk about what respectful, accountable, and professional attitudes and behaviors look like.

The 10% Downright Ugly Attitudes

Some staff members have a great need for order, predictability, and control. They prefer to follow specific routines, work with their chosen group of individuals, and take breaks at the same time no matter what. Organizational change can pose a huge threat to these nurses, who function reasonably well in a stable environment. No matter how many explanations or how much time they have had to digest the change process, they will never accept what is going on. They will not change! Nurse managers will spend an inordinate amount of time trying to convince, cajole, and influence their behavior. It will not work!

MISERY LOVES COMPANY

Nurses with miserable attitudes need company to fuel their fire and are expert at recruiting a following. Their attitude often reflects pride in holding steadfast to the "old ways," refusing to accept change, and seeing themselves as purists (real nurses). They can stir up all kinds of issues in the workplace pot. They do their best work behind the scenes, when the nurse manager is out of sight. In some cases, they are seen, especially by physicians, to be "a terrific nurse"—the epitome of efficiency and excellence.

A TOUGH CHALLENGE

Despite the fact that some nurses do not support the direction in which the practice setting is heading, those with ugly attitudes often refuse to leave or transfer. They hang on, convinced that "things will get back to normal." Some have very little insight into how their attitude is affecting their colleagues or patient care. Others, who are close to retirement, have a sense of entitlement and believe that their attitude is not a problem. It is "just the way I am." When this attitude prevails, other staff members learn to work around them and will even defend or make excuses for their behavior.

Downright ugly behaviors present nurse managers with huge personal and professional challenges that can test the manager to the point where he/she may want to leave! In the end, however, after being managed from a performance perspective, some nurses with toxic behaviors may have to leave. They lack either the self-awareness or the desire to "improve" their attitude. If these individuals are not managed, they along with their cohorts will ultimately threaten the quality of care and the ability of staff to thrive.

Fast facts in a nutshell

- Message to staff: Attitude is a choice. Choose wisely!
- Message to self: I cannot be responsible for changing staff members' attitudes: I can only create the conditions and hope that will help individuals reflect and choose an attitude that helps them to thrive.

THE BOTTOM LINE

Staff members are responsible for the attitude they choose. When they choose behaviors that reflect toxic attitudes, they must be held accountable within the context of their Standards of Practice. Nurse managers are ultimately responsible and accountable for helping staff manage their behaviors. For both you and your staff, managing attitudes is both difficult and uncomfortable, but it is mandatory for the sake of quality care and healthy interpersonal relationships.

PROFILING UGLY ATTITUDES AMONG A GROUP OF CHARACTERS

It is fair to say that the following "characters" are but a few typically found in most workplaces. Everyone will admit that their behavior creates strains on workplace relationships and can distract others from patient care activities. The following three demonstrate some of the most commonly found ugly attitudes in the workplace. The degree of distress they cause is considered mild to moderate. As their manager, count yourself among the fortunate if you have only one. In many cases all three may be present.

Negaholics

What they do:
These individuals are chronically negative. They are predisposed to whine and complain about just about anything. Nothing is ever good enough, and no amount of jumping through hoops to please them or brighten their mood will put a smile on their faces. For example, as the new shift comes on duty, the "negaholic" will greet them with, "We had a rough night, and you are going to have a terrible day! Bye!"

Another favorite behavior is repetitive complaining and whining about the same issue. When asked what they plan to do about the situation, the response is usually silence. Or, they will say, "I don't know, it's not my job to figure it out."

Whining and complaining is a symptom of an unexpressed feeling or need. The problem is that other nurses admit that "negaholics" have to power to propel them into a negative mindset.

What they may want: Attention, recognition, personal power, help.

What they don't want: To improve the situation.

What you can do:

- Try to identify what they are *not* saying.
  DO NOT UNDER ANY CIRCUMSTANCE BECOME THEIR PSYCHOTHERAPIST!
- Be careful about how you offer help. When you ask, "How can I help you" (to correct your bad behavior), your unspoken message is, "You may not be capable of helping yourself, therefore you need me to help you." When you take responsibility for the behavior of your staff members, you take away their power to help themselves. They then have an excuse to defer their responsibility; it gets them off the hook. Instead, point out their behavior and ask them how it affects quality of care and their peer relationships. Point out that this behavior is inconsistent with a professional practice environment, and ask what think they can do to improve their behavior. Help them to develop a plan for managing their behavior. Express confidence in their ability to create a positive outcome.
- Engage all staff in conversations about which behaviors strengthen workplace relationships and which do not. Reinforce your professional conduct expectations of all staff.
- Be prepared to go down the performance road if chronic negativity persists.

Rumor and Gossip Mongers

What they do:

These staff members have the dirt on everyone and love to share what they know with anyone who will listen. The research community has not yet weighed in about the effects of workplace gossip. Some say "good gossip" is a positive relational tool used by women to strengthen connectedness. However, in some workplaces, staff members frequently describe the hurtful effects of gossip because it threatens harmony. They also express discomfort when approached by someone with a "juicy bit about someone else." Once again, individuals are inclined to respond with silence for fear of compromising their relationships or because they do not know how to manage the behavior.

What you can do:
- Ask yourself why individuals keep hurtful gossip alive and well, even though most would like it to stop.
- Ask staff what gossip does for them and what it may be masking.
- Recognize that gossip is a complex issue that may relate to power and control issues in the workplace.
- Ask yourself and staff, "What situations in the workplace lead us to feel powerless?"
- Help staff to look at and name the situations that create feelings of powerlessness, and facilitate discussion about how to handle the situations differently.
- Invite further conversations about how staff can strengthen positive personal and professional power.

Houseplants

What they do:
These individuals have an incredible knack for doing as little as possible. They sit on a chair for most of the shift, manag-

ing to avoid answering call bells, the telephone, or inquiries. Everyone knows their game, yet few will ever say anything. Meanwhile, staff resentment builds. If a staff member makes a comment, it is usually humorous and ultimately futile. Houseplants are expert at ignoring dirty looks and subtle rebukes. Nurses feel that they are doing the Houseplant's work in addition to their own and will wonder why the manager is not doing anything about this nurse at a time when staffing is tight and every pair of hands needed.

Sometimes Houseplants are worn out and unaware that they are not doing their share of the work. Sometimes they are lazy! When they lack the insight and feel unable to do the work they were hired to do, they are not living up to the requirements of their professional contract. If there is a medical reason, nurse managers must help these nurses come to the realization that they may require medical attention. If their behavior is linked to attitude, your challenge is greater. It becomes a performance issue that cannot be ignored. In addressing the situation head on, you provide welcome relief for the nurse who is not sharing the load and his/her peers who are angrier than hornets! A potential win-win situation develops for all.

What you can do:
- Be there! If you are not, you cannot know what is really going on.
- Every once in awhile, cruise through your workplace and observe the "flow" of activity to see who is doing what, who is out there with the patients, and who is sitting behind the desk.

- Look for patterns of activity among staff (i.e., who responds to call bells, phone calls, etc.).
- If you suspect a Houseplant in your midst, it is your job to uproot them!
- Meet with the staff person to point out your observations, the practice implications, and listen for an explanation. Ask about his/her plan to remedy the situation.
- State your expectations for improved performance and schedule a follow-up meeting.

Fast facts in a nutshell: summary

- Managing attitudes is essential for creating healthy workplace relationships.
- Healthy workplace relationships grow happy staff.
- Happy staff stays.

Chapter 12

Got Queens, Princesses, and Workplace Terrorists?

Managing Their Reign of Terror

INTRODUCTION

"Queen" behavior in the workplace is not unique to nursing. However, in a predominantly female workplace, feelings of powerlessness exist. Such conditions can foster the emergence of particularly aggressive behaviors attributed to the presence of a Workplace Queen. This chapter describes one of the most toxic workplace behaviors and its serious impact on staff relationships and quality of worklife. Overt and covert operations for managing workplace terrorist behavior are revealed.

In this chapter, you will learn:

1. To identify toxic behaviors in the practice setting.
2. Tips for dethroning workplace queens and managing a toxic workplace.

WORKPLACE TERRORISM UNCOVERED

The use of the terms "terror" and "terrorism" may seem extreme descriptors of workplace behavior, but their impact can be devastating to individuals, demoralizing to entire staffs, and damaging to the reputations of organizations. The good news is that only a very small percentage of nurses ever become "queens" of workplace terrorism. Many Queens are unaware of their damaging Queen behavior, while others are acutely aware and choose to use their informal negative power to hurt their colleagues. Queens are tough to manage (especially in a unionized environment). Many nurse managers can become victims of a Queen when engaged in a power struggle. In a few of the worst case scenarios, Queens and their princesses deliberately set out to "destroy" any nurse manager who gets in their way, and the rate of turnover of nurse managers in a toxic practice setting becomes the lore of legends. Battles against a manager can be so psychologically fierce and physically draining that managers are unable to do their jobs and eventually leave rather than continue the struggle.

Workplace Queens are the embodiment of toxicity of the worst kind, and their behavior is nothing short of bullying. Although the topic of bullying is discussed in Chapter 13, Queens deserve their own chapter because of their looming presence and prominence in our nursing culture. Almost every nurse will encounter a Queen at least once in their career. These Queens may appear to be the "best" nurses on the unit. They are well versed in "how things are done around here" and generally have a great deal of experience. They do their best work and their most damage where and when detection is least likely.

The impact of the Queen's toxic behavior is not limited to the practice setting and can leech into other areas of the organization, community, and beyond.

AN OVERVIEW OF KINGS AND QUEENS

The counterparts of Queens and Princesses are, of course, Kings and Princes. The presence of a Queen/King and their followers can seriously undermine efforts to recruit and retain staff. In nursing, there are likely to be more Queens than Kings because of the larger number of women in the profession. Although this chapter focuses on Queens and Princesses, it does not mean that males are exempt from similarly poor behavior.

Gender usually determines how the toxic behaviors play out in the workplace. Recent research on women's patterns of relating, managing anger, and bullying provides valuable insight into the Queen's behavior. The culture of nursing is ripe for Queen behavior, as evident in nursing's old adage, "Everyone knows we eat our young!," that has lingered far too long. Workplace Queens thrive because of nurses' proclivities for stable relationships. They do not want to cause trouble, so they maintain a culture of silence. Queens exist because they can. Nursing's tacit acceptance of Queens and fear of dealing with them must end if nursing hopes to retain and recruit staff. Although tongue-in-cheek humor is used to bring this subject into the light of day, Queen behavior is no laughing matter. Using the famous words of Dr. Phil, "You can't change what you don't acknowledge," nursing must take a long hard look at a profession that permits nurses to hurt one another.

The practice must end through reflection, examination, education and meaningful change.

QUEENS AND THEIR COURTIERS

Queens have great power in the workplace that often allows them to supplant the role of the nurse manager. Their power lies in their ability to create a following in the workplace, inspire loyalty, and engage other staff in actions considered detrimental to healthy team relationships. The Queen's followers are known as "princesses," "wanna' be's," or "queens in training." They often mimic the behaviors of the Queen, but generally do not possess the same degree of power.

Fast facts in a nutshell

- The toxic impact of queen behavior is compounded when others are called to court.
- Some go willingly while others join out of fear of becoming the next target.

PROFILES OF WORKPLACE ROYALTY

Queens and Princesses employ a number of tactics to maintain their position and power. Without the benefit of psychoanalysis, it is difficult to speculate on their motivation. Why do individuals who profess they are caring resort to soul-destroying behavior? Some say it is typical of oppressed group behavior, while others conclude that it is misplaced or misdirected anger. Another interpretation suggest these behaviors mask feelings of anxiety related to a changing workplace, a strong desire to maintain the status quo, fear of the unknown, or a high, even pathological, need for power and control. The following examples illustrate a few preferred tactics.

Intimidation: The Queen Is Not Amused!

A typical scenario plays out as follows.

- A staff nurse returns from break and is met by the icy stare of the Queen, who is standing in the hallway staring first at her watch, then glaring at the nurse, then back at her watch, and then back to the nurse. She is silent as she delivers the final "if looks could kill" nonverbal blow! Without speaking, the Queen has accomplished an act of intimidation designed to make the nurse feel any number of emotions including:
  - Guilt: for being perceived as late when she/he probably was not.
  - Fear: of being watched.
  - Anger: at being embarrassed in front of others.
  - Resentful at being treated as a child.
  - Anxious: about what may happen next.

Over time, these negative emotions build up inside individuals and groups. If not managed, they create secondary issues, including illness, avoidance, and breakdowns in communication that impair team functioning and patient care. To prevent repeated victimization, the nurse may call in sick, change his or her clinical assignments, and keep communication to a bare minimum.

Blaming Others: Off with Their Heads!

Queens have a knack for blaming others and rarely accept responsibility for their own behavior. Nothing is ever the fault of the Queen. If you are waiting for insight to occur, it may never happen. Despite great efforts to help, some staff's personalities never accept responsibility for their actions.

Ridiculing Others: Peasants Be Gone!

A favorite tactic is to use an imperious tone of voice with young graduates. The goal is to disempower a nurse with a remark such as, "You don't know that? Everyone knows that!" Or, "What *did* they teach you in school anyway?"

Disappearing Others: You See Me, but I Choose Not to See You!

In the presence of the Queens and Princesses, the victim is treated as invisible. For example, if a nurse on the target list walks into a room where the Queen and princesses are holding court, that nurse is completely ignored. The Queen makes no eye contact whatsoever and avoids directing any remarks to the individual or acknowledging his/her presence.

Public Floggings: A Power Boosting Moment!

Being told, "That's stupid!" or "Don't be ridiculous!" diminishes self-worth and destabilizes self-confidence. This behavior may eventually shut people down to the point where they are filled with self-doubt, lose confidence in their ability to do their job, and become ill.

Exclusionary Tactics: So You are Not on the 'A' List? Too Bad, So Sad!

Certain staff members may be deliberately excluded from social occasions. The buzz intensifies as courtiers speculate about "why?" Another tactic is to inform new staff members not to use the regular staff refrigerator to store their lunches until they come off the "probationary period."

DETHRONING WORKPLACE KINGS AND QUEENS

Managing Queen behavior is never optional. How it is managed depends on the type of behavior, the circumstances, the experience of the manager, and the resources available to support the process.

Queen behavior will not thrive in practice environments where:

- There is a requirement for adherence to Nursing Practice Standards.
- Nurse managers possesses self-awareness and strong leadership skills.
- The focus is on patient/client-centered care.
- There are opportunities for staff development.
- Respectful behavior is required in the workplace.
- Staff receive regular performance feedback

Fast facts in a nutshell

- Dethroning workplace Queens and Kings is never optional.
- Declare the buffet closed by saying, "Nurses will no longer eat their young!"

SPECIAL OPS TACTICS FOR NURSE MANAGERS

To tackle Queen behavior in your workplace, use both short- and long term strategies.

Short-Term Strategies

1. First take care of yourself: conduct a self-assessment (your readiness to deal with a very tough problem).
2. Write down what you know about the behavior. Determine the level of impact and develop a plan.
3. Schedule a meeting with the Queen to discuss the issue(s). Be prepared for a sick call or excuse and the potential for endless delays. Avoid allowing this ploy to drag on (the Queen's strategy is to wait you out).
4. Conduct the first meeting according to your performance management protocols. Point out the inappropriate behaviors. Identify your expectations for conduct.
5. Link the Queen behaviors to the Standards of Practice that govern professional relationships and accountability.
6. Keep the meeting short (no more than 20 minutes—this coveys a message that you are in charge).
7. Express your confidence that behavior will change and schedule check-in meetings.
8. Expect a sick call or a doctor's note identifying a need for short- or long-term sick leave. Stay on top of the situation and modify your plan.

Long-Term Strategies

1. Schedule lunch-and-learn sessions or staff meetings that include conversations about the following.
   - Living the value of respect in our workplace,
   - Providing feedback to our colleagues in our Professional Practice Settings.

- Bullying in the workplace.
- Accountability in healthy workplace relationships.

2. Consult with other nurse managers about their approach to managing Queen behaviors.
3. Periodically ask staff members about professionalism in the workplace and what it looks like.
4. Create opportunities for assertiveness training.
5. Consult with other departments about becoming strategic in preventing and managing this type of behavior.

Fast facts in a nutshell: summary

- Queen behavior is not exclusive to nursing.
- Queens thrive because they can.
- Terrorism in the workplace cannot thrive when there is strong, effective leadership in a practice setting driven by the Standards of Professional Practice.

Chapter 13

Got Bullying?

Managing the Sound of Silence

INTRODUCTION

The phenomenon of bullying in nursing is not new. Yet despite policies of zero tolerance, bullying continues as an "organizational undiscussable" (Beer & Eisenstadt, 2000) that incubates in a culture of silence. Dealing with a workplace bully who is a nurse presents the nurse manager with time-consuming and extraordinary personal and professional challenges. This chapter focuses less on the troubling characteristics of bullies and more on what to do about them. The intent is to encourage you to take the necessary steps to support and fuel your resolve to rid your workplace of bullying behaviors.

In this chapter, you will learn:

1. Bullying is preventable.

2. You vital role in eliminating bullying from the practice setting.
3. Skills and processes for managing bullying.

THE BEGINNING OF THE END
OF WORKPLACE BULLYING IN NURSING

Ten years ago, the existence of bullying in nursing and health-care organizations was well known but rarely talked about. Nurse managers and staff were reluctant or unsure how to characterize this behavior. Even more important, they were unsure how to deal with it. Managers who attempted to tackle the issue met with little organizational support. The presence of a bully was either tolerated in silence or victimized staff members left "to further advance their careers." Remaining staff would tippy-toe around the bully, excusing their actions with, "You get used to it," or "They don't really mean anything by it. She/he is a really good nurse." Even with the advent of the highly touted organizational zero tolerance policies, bullying flourished and continues to this day. **The fact that bullying is still prevalent illustrates that current strategies are not working.**

With the onset of massive organizational change, workplace conditions of powerlessness, fear of the unknown, and frustration, nurses increasingly turn on one another. **The bottom line: Bullying must stop!** It drives new nurses out of the profession, causes experienced nurses to work around a colleague, and makes other staff ill. As daunting as it may seem, nurse managers have the greatest ability to end bullying in clinical practice settings.

MONKEY IN THE MIDDLE

In unionized environments, nurse managers who attempt to manage a bully can be set up for a "monkey in the middle" situation. They become caught between the perpetually warring factions of union and management, where the process can erode into an attack on the manager's credibility.

ARE YOU UP FOR THE CHALLENGE?

Before dealing with a bully, many nurse managers will quietly ask themselves if they are "up for the challenge." Some believe that they may "be hung out to dry" and will search their souls asking if sacrificing their mental health is too high a price to pay. Some may ask if the situation is really all that bad. Others may believe that if they didn't witness it, they cannot do anything about it. A few may even excuse the behavior and justify it with a "well that's just the way they are." The cost of excuses and inaction is high, and other staff will pay the price. You will lose the respect of staff; staff will live and work in a state of fear; and deep inside you will know that you are not doing the right thing. In the end, good staff members will be left to manage a struggle that should not be theirs in the first place, and the bully will retain the seat of power.

WHY BULLIES THRIVE

Despite knowing a great deal about workplace bullies, what makes them tick, their impact on victims, peers, quality of care, and costs to the organization, they continue to exist. Why? Because they can! We tolerate bullying behavior because:

1. Bullies are scary! Many nurse managers are also afraid of the bully.
2. Managers may deny the existence of a bully in *their* workplace.
3. There may be a lack of meaningful policies or support for nurse managers.
4. Managers may fear or lack time to go down that long and winding road of performance management.
5. There is a fear of escalating the behavior into physical violence.
6. There is a fear of an adversarial encounter with the union or litigious actions by the staff member.
7. There is a reluctance to hop on the medical leave of absence merry-go-round, where stressed staff members take medically approved sick leave, come back, go off again, and return ad infinitum!
8. There is a fear of the consequences of more work on your already heavy workload.

NOT FOR THE FAINT OF HEART

Given the energy crisis that most of us are experiencing in today's workplaces, many nurse managers shake their heads in despair at the thought of a staff member who bullies. Many will wearily declare, "I don't have the time or the energy for this [expletive deleted]." Not having the time is not an option.

The implications of not managing bullying behavior are far reaching and include:

1. **The obvious**
   - Staff will leave.
   - Care will suffer.
   - Sick time will increase.
   - Morale will tank.
   - Bullies hold onto their power.
2. **The less obvious**
   - Bullying *is* unprofessional conduct.
   - Managers cannot (by virtue of their Standards of Practice) turn a blind eye to unprofessional conduct.
   - Bullying violates Standards of Practice and undermines the nursing Code of Ethics.
   - You are leading a workplace that may be driven by fear (generated by the bully).
   - This 1% (the bully) of your staff is holding at least 99% psychologically hostage!
   - You will lose the respect of your staff.
   - The word on the street will be, "Don't work there."

Fast facts in a nutshell

- Nurse managers hold the most power organizationally and professionally to manage bullying behavior.
- Nurse managers are ultimately accountable for managing bullying in the workplace.

"THE SECRET" TO FINDING COURAGE

The secret is to adopt the attitude, "It's not personal; it's professional." Your leadership ensures that patients receive nursing care delivered by competent professionals in a healing and safe practice environment. Your job is to ensure that this happens. There is no compromising when your standards require you to take action!

PRACTICE STANDARDS MATTER

When workplace bullies run amok, professional nursing practice becomes embroiled in, and distracted by, unhealthy and destructive relationships. In managing bullying behavior, nurse managers send the following messages.

1. As nurses, we are duty and legally bound by our Standards of Practice.
2. Each registered nurse is accountable for his/her practice.
3. Untoward behavior (unprofessional conduct) is inconsistent with nursing Professional Standards and cannot be tolerated.

According to the Practice Standards for nurse leaders, a key accountability is to ensure that staff complies with Practice Standards. **By linking bullying behavior to Nursing Practice Standards, bullying becomes a noncompliant and unacceptable behavior.** With full knowledge of the standards and their applications, the employment contract, appropriate organizational resources, and the right attitude and skill mix, nurse managers have the tools to eliminate bullying in the workplace.

A THREE-TIERED APPROACH TO MANAGING BULLIES

Self

- Once you identify bullying behavior in your practice area, reflect on your feelings about the situation (i.e., are you afraid of the bully, is your workload leaving you feel overwhelmed, are you ready to take this on?). Get a grip on your own situation before dealing with the bullying behavior.

If you witness bullying behavior:

- First gather your thoughts and record observations, including dates and times;
- Plan your approach to meet, discuss, and create desired outcomes.
- Inform your boss and Human Resources Department (if appropriate) that you are about to tackle suspected bullying behavior, giving them a heads up about your approach, your short- and long-term plans, and your anticipated outcome.
- Seek support from a trusted colleague for role playing in preparation for your conversation with the bully.
- Get a good night's sleep before the meeting.
- If the person (bully) has anger management issues, take this into consideration.
- Keep the meeting brief (15–20 minutes).

If you are aware of, but have not witnessed, the bullying incident:

- Don your Sherlock Holmes hat, perform your investigative homework, conduct a self-check, and begin the process of eliminating this destructive force.
- Assign priority status to managing this unprofessional conduct.
- Remind yourself that you must follow through with this action or staff morale and patient care will continue to suffer.
- Gather and record your facts: observations, time, dates, and presence of others.
- Give a "heads up" to the person to whom you report.
- Schedule an appointment with the staff member.
- Before you meet, get a good night's sleep.
- Repeat the mantra, "It is not personal; it is professional."
- Develop a small support network or recruit a colleague to practice your feedback session before you meet with the staff person.
- Proceed according to performance management protocols.
- At the beginning of the meeting, explain to the nurse that part of your professional administrative accountability lies in managing situations that may adversely affect quality of patient care and workplace relationships .
- Describe your observations, listen to feedback, and help the staff develop a plan for the remedial process.

Staff

- You have the administrative and professional responsibility for determining the impact of bullying behavior on staff and taking steps to reestablish harmony in the workplace. In doing so, you create a healing environment and a healthy workplace where people want to work.
- Most staff members know about and hope that you will deal with the workplace bully. The irony is that for obvious reasons of confidentiality, they will never know what steps you take to curb the bullying behavior. You can, however, send a subtle yet powerful message that healthy workplaces are mandatory for the provision of quality care and that every staff member is vital to the process. Henceforth, you will all strive to create a workplace where nurses want to work.
- You can begin with a "back-to-basics" conversation about what is vital to healthy workplace relationships and practice. Follow this with a plan to achieve the goal. Staff will quietly be reassured about who is in control and appreciate that the element of fear is no longer tolerated in the workplace.
- Look for opportunities every day to connect Standards with day-to-day relationships and nursing practice.

Organization

- Raise awareness if zero tolerance policies are not embedded in the organization, and challenge the management structure to take a deeper look at why they are not working.

- Recommend a forum for other nurse managers to discuss the realities of managing professional practice, including its underbelly.
- Identify further organizational supports and learning needs for effective management of bullying behavior.

Fast facts in a nutshell: summary

- Managing bullying behavior is a professional responsibility and an act of courage. You can do it! You must do it!

Part IV

Predicting Your
Workplace Future
Create It! Manage It! Love It!

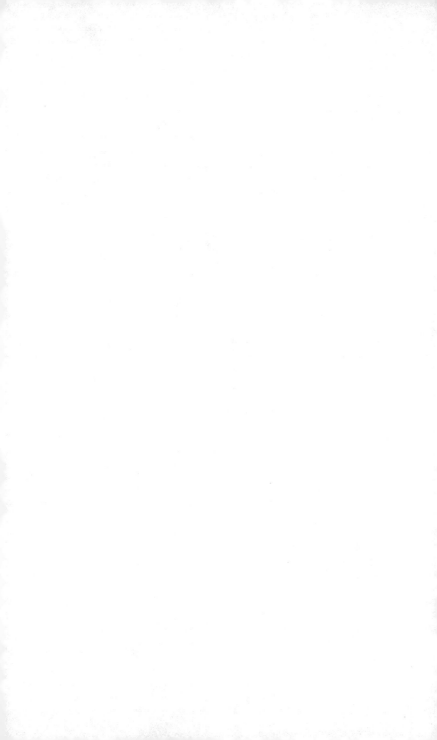

Chapter 14

Mission Impossible?

Managing Work-Life Balance

INTRODUCTION

Generations X and Y have it right! Unlike their parents, they expect to achieve balance at home and at work. Nurse managers are keenly aware of the conflict that exists in achieving this balance, particularly because nurses have a deeply embedded work ethic that includes self-sacrifice. How do you lead by example and facilitate individual achievement of work-life balance? This chapter will help you to recognize the signs of imbalance, how to course correct your staff, and how to model a new and "balanced" you.

In this chapter, you will learn:

1. The impact of a "brushfire management" style on work-life balance.
2. The necessity for change.
3. Tips for completing your mission.

THE PROBLEM

During the 1990s, when downsizing, restructuring, and massive lays-offs were the norm, nurse managers were catapulted into a maelstrom of leadership and operational situations that traditional styles of management could not resolve. In their struggle to adapt, many nurse managers unwittingly adopted a "brushfire management" style that for many has become a way of life. Although unlikely to be found in the management literature, this style is highly popular. Borne out of necessity, it practiced on a daily basis and is a major threat to work-life balance.

Brushfire management occurs when busy managers are constantly trying to "put out fires." Days consist of managing countless and often scattered day-to-day operational issues, responding to organizational demands, and trying to resolve one crisis before another erupts. As a result, many managers feel mentally and physically exhausted, inadequate to the job, and guilty about things "left undone." If that were not enough, the situation replicates itself when the nurse manager goes home to meet the demands of family living and community membership.

REFLECTION: ARE YOU A "BRUSHFIRE MANAGER"?

You are if you demonstrate some of the following behaviors.

- Your wristwatch has 25 or more hours a day.
- You feel stressed most or all of the time.

- You usually arrive at work with wet hair.
- You ain't got no satisfaction.
- You are related to Alice's March hare and are frequently heard to mutter, "I'm late, I'm late for a very important (meeting)."
- You have forgotten how to say "no."
- Your office weathered a tornado last year (at least that is your story and you are sticking to it), scattering papers everywhere, and you still have not had time to tidy your office.
- You feel like a mouse running on a treadmill and a puppet on a string.
- Guilt is your new "BFF" (Best Friend Forever!).
- You return to work after hours to "finish up" or fill a U-haul with paperwork to take home.

Fast facts in a nutshell

- Work-life balance occurs when you effectively manage your responsibilities at work, at home, and in your community, leaving you with a sense of emotional and physical well-being.
- It is not about being all things to all people.

A NOTE ABOUT WHIRLING DERVISH SYNDROME

If you are prone to a brushfire management style, you are at risk of succumbing to chronic "whirling dervish syndrome."

If you have any of the following symptoms, burnout is a hair's breadth away. Your symptoms may include:

- A foreboding sense of neverending challenges.
- You feel as if you are spinning in random circles.
- You believe you are going nowhere fast.
- You suffer from fatigue.
- You multitask by talking on two cell phones at the same time, with your call waiting on hold as you gather notes for a meeting.
- You walk away from someone while they are still talking to you.

If allowed to go unchecked, your physical and mental health may suffer, workplace relationships will deteriorate, burnout will be a step away, and regret will be profound. And the question that begs an answer is, "Who will lead your staff if you are unable to lead yourself and demonstrate balance at work and at home?"

WHEN BRUSHFIRE MANAGEMENT INTERFERES WITH YOUR PERSONAL LIFE

The following situations are all too common when work spills over into your personal life.

- You forget to pick your child up from piano lessons.
- You miss your daughter's soccer game.
- You take a leisurely bubble bath with your "Crackberry" to answer e-mails.

- You have no "me" time.
- Sex or sleep? Sex or sleep? You choose sleep.
- You are unable to participate in family events because you have "work to do."
- You allow "guilt" to follow you home from work.
- Your pets run for cover when you arrive home.
- You yell at your houseplants!

YOUR MISSION: TO SEEK AND ESTABLISH BALANCE AT WORK, AT HOME, AND IN YOUR COMMUNITY

Should you choose to accept, **your mission is to embark on a journey of personal change**, to capture the essence of a state of well-being at home, at work, and as a member of community, and to model, lead, and inspire your staff to do the same.

In Accepting Your Mission

1. Accept that if you keep doing what you've always done, you'll keep getting what you always got (Thank you Dr. Phil!)
2. Engage in self-reflection to increase your understanding of why brushfire management has such a grip on you.
3. Be willing to engage in new learning.
4. Accept that it is okay to try new ways of being, fail, and try again.

If You Refuse to Accept This Mission

The risks of not accepting change puts you and your staff in survival, as opposed to thriving, mode. It places all of you on a slippery personal and professional slope. Some of the dangers that you may face if you refuse your mission include:

- Physical problems associated with not taking care of yourself. These include fatigue, mental and physical illness, and burnout.
- Emotional problems associated with pushing feelings aside, as you and your staff struggle with multiple demands. When you fail to reflect on your situation and feelings, you run the risk of increasing frustration, anger, resentment, and powerlessness that can lead to toxic attitudes and behaviors.
- Potential for increased absenteeism, sick time, and an inability to recruit and retain.
- Complaints of "alienation of affection" from colleagues, family, and friends.

The best hope that you and your staff have for achieving work-life balance is for you to take the lead and inspire your staff to follow.

Fast facts in a nutshell

- The best way to achieve personal and professional work-life balance is to commit to change, take the lead

> in changing your behavior, and inspire your staff to follow.
> - In the short term, change is difficult; in the long term, you may wonder, "Why did I wait so long?"

TIPS FOR COMPLETING YOUR MISSION

These tips work in all settings whether it is home, at work, or in the community.

1. Just say "no."
Easier said than done. Sometimes we must question our motives. What are the benefits and consequences of saying "no"? Wise words from an unknown source advise that we should "Never do anything for someone else that they are perfectly capable of doing for themselves."

2. Reflect on and realign your priorities.
Is it essential that *you* do laundry every day? How is work distributed at home and at work? Does it really matter that your children do not miter their corners when making their beds? What are the relationship costs of insisting that your home be on the Junior League Christmas at Home tours?

3. Nurture relationships with your colleagues, friends, and family.
When you find yourself caught up in brushfire management, it is easy to focus on the tasks and lose sight of the people in your life. We are vulnerable to taking others for granted until

faced with the stunning reality that one day they may not be there when we really need them. Remember the old saying, "No one on their deathbed was ever thanked for staying late at the office."

4. Create "me" time.
Creating "me" time is for some an almost impossible task. Women, in particular, are often guilt ridden if they take time away from perceived responsibilities. They view this as an act of selfishness. Family members question how they will survive when you are "off-limits." No matter what, resist the temptation to return to your old patterns of behavior. Like any other art form, this new you process takes practice and patience.

5. Actively reduce the number of demands you place on yourself.
"When all else fails, lower your standards (source unknown)." While you may shudder at the thought, think about this: In today's changing and complex workplaces, everyone is on a learning curve and super humans are still in the cloning phase.

6. Lighten up.
Laughter is good medicine. Whether you are at home or at work, rediscovering your sense of humor is a powerful tool in establishing work-life balance. Humor is a natural and therapeutic tool of nurses and an important aspect of our nursing culture. Use it or lose it!

7. Reframe negative situations.
Look for opportunities and possibilities. Focus on positive change.

8. Leave your Blackberry and other devices at home while on vacation.

Consider office e-mails off limits while on vacation. If your mind is at the office when you are on a beach, you are not in true vacation mode and are living a lie. If the thought of being PD free causes palpitations, change is no longer optional. You need help!

YOU: A WORK IN PROGRESS

Achieving work-life balance is an individual, personal, and professional issue that can have serious implications if left unresolved. Deciding to change and then inspiring change within and among your staff members requires a willingness and commitment to "try on new behaviors" aimed at creating a sense of well-being, enhancing performance, and creating healthier workplace relationships. If you have not done so already, start now by giving yourself permission to consider yourself a "work in progress" and see what unfolds. Invite staff to join you on your journey. Call a staff meeting to discover what factors in your environment promote or inhibit work-life balance and what can be done to achieve it. Periodically check with staff to see how well you are doing, create opportunities to exchange ideas, and acknowledge and celebrate successes.

Fast facts in a nutshell: summary

- It is easy to talk about work-life balance, but harder to "walk the talk."
- Staff members will watch your every move to see if you really mean what you say.
- For your own sake and the health of your staff, if you want to achieve work-life balance, you go first!

Chapter 15

Creating Your Future

Managing Purposeful and Values-Driven Workplace Relationships

INTRODUCTION

In a world of renewed economic downturns and layoffs, nurse managers must be crystal clear about the value-added role their service offers in the provision of quality care and excellence in practice. Equally important is that staff members be clear about their value as individuals and as a group of professionals in healthcare service delivery. This chapter discusses the importance of establishing your own workplace mission, vision, and values statements separate from, but complementary to, the organization's. The chapter also discusses ways to bring them to life and live them every day in practice and in all your workplace relationships.

In this chapter, you will learn:

1. The value of creating your own practice setting's mission, vision, and values.
2. The importance of trust in the workplace and workplace charters.
3. Tips for becoming a trustworthy nurse manager.

PREDICT YOUR WORKPLACE FUTURE: CREATE YOUR MISSION, VISION, AND VALUES

Peter Drucker said, "The best way to predict the future is to create it." What kind of workplace future do you want? What does staff want? These questions are normally not asked or answered by nurse managers and their staffs; they usually default to the organizational culture's formal statements about "Our Mission, Vision, and Values" generated by senior leadership at a strategic planning retreat.

WHEN STAFF LOOK BUT DO NOT SEE

Typically, nurse managers are expected to disseminate and discuss the organizational mission, vision, and values (M,V,V) statements and secure "buy-in" from their staffs to the future direction of the organization. Staff members respond, in turn, with cynical and tacit approval, without ever truly owning the words or their intended message. The reason is that most have witnessed countless violations of newly minted organizational mission, vision, and values statements. The stories of leaders "not walking the talk" are legendary. **Too often, staff members are treated badly in organizations where "people are our greatest assets."** They become disillusioned with the breakdown of decision-making processes and practices that give way to dysfunctional organizational power and politics. In the minds of many, the mission, vision, and values are meaningless.

Fast facts in a nutshell

• Most staff members have a vague recollection that somewhere in their organization is a laminated plaque depicting the organizational mission, vision, and values statements that are doomed to suffer a lonely existence. They are destined to hang between the elevators for everyone to see without really seeing.

WHAT WE ALL WANT

Fundamentally, **most staff members want and need to have meaningful work,** contribute to the greater good, and know that they matter and make a difference in service to others. When this happens, they provide better care, achieve personal and professional power, and demonstrate healthier and collegial workplace relationships. When they develop their own practice setting, mission, vision, and values statements that complement the larger organizational M,V,V, they are creating a framework or a blueprint that guides the quality of their worklife, their relationships, and the actions for achieving excellence in service provision.

CREATING YOUR PRACTICE SETTINGS MISSION, VISION, AND VALUES

Especially during times of chaos and change, nurse managers need to help staff connect the work in their practice setting to the overall purpose of the organization. Unit-based missions, vision, and values serve as a "closer to home" and complementary subset to that of the broader organization.

Fast facts in a nutshell

- Practice setting mission, vision, and values statements provide staff with a sense of direction, create context for the type of care/service delivered in the practice setting, and reinforce the moral and ethical drivers that guide the decisions and actions of the healthcare team.

A **mission** describes the purpose of a clinical program or service and aligns staff on a shared journey.

A **vision** reflects "our hopes for a preferred future" (Oakley & Krug, 1994, p. 227).

Values represent the ethical and moral standards that will guide professional care and relationships in a practice setting.

WHERE TO START

1. Create opportunities to promote reflection and dialogue that provide staff with an opportunity to create a vision of how the members see themselves and the role they play in service delivery. Try asking some of the following questions. Record the discussion and use the answers in your planning your vision statement.
    - Why do we exist as a practice setting? What is our shared purpose in the provision of healthcare service delivery? Why are we different?
    - Why is this service essential to overall organizational success? What business are we in? (Do not accept answers such as, "Because we care for mothers and children or because we care for surgical patients.")
    - What special roles do our various team members play in the provision of care?
2. Reflect on and discuss the professional attributes and scopes of practice with all staff.
3. Engage staff in the "Postcard from Home" exercise (see Appendix A).
4. Conduct a Values Development exercise (Appendix B).
5. Have a conversation about "Living Our Values" (Appendix C).
6. Have fun with the "Back to Our Future Exercise (Appendix D).
7. Use the Back to the Future Discussion Guide to help staff identify specific suggestions for improving quality of worklife or strengthening workplace relationships (Appendix E).
8. Review your Mission, Vision, and Values annually.

BUILD TRUST, AND THEY WILL COME

Trust building is the relational glue for interpersonal relationships. It determines how well staff members work together. Nurses know how to build and maintain trust within the context of the professional and therapeutic relationship to achieve successful patient/client care outcomes. Trust is an equally important quality aspect of healthy workplace relationships. In many of today's chaotic and changing workplaces, trust at an interpersonal and organizational level is at an all-time low. Without trust in the nurse manager, the practice setting metaphorically becomes a rudderless ship. **Without trust in staff members and their abilities, nurse managers cannot effectively lead.**

TRUST IN THE WORKPLACE

Trust is a complex and multilevel attribute. It is about integrity, honesty, transparency, and accountability, the essence of which is captured in Nursing's Standards of Professional Practice.

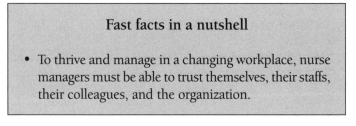

Fast facts in a nutshell

- To thrive and manage in a changing workplace, nurse managers must be able to trust themselves, their staffs, their colleagues, and the organization.

Trust in Self

When relationships and work processes are muddied by negative interpersonal relationships, organizational politics, and constant change, trust in self is challenged. Under the constant scrutiny of staff's watchful eyes, **it is vital that nurse managers model trust in self.** Nurse managers who do what they say they will do are transparent in their actions and conversations, inspire staff to do the right thing, and speak to organizational issues that influence quality of care and quality of worklife create an environment of high trust.

Trust in Staff

Some nurse managers believe trust must be earned, while others believe that individuals are worthy of trust until they prove otherwise. Being willing to trust staff up front:

- Leaves the door open for mutual trust building.
- Inspires accountability.
- Implies that it is okay to take a leap of faith, try new things, and make appropriate independent decisions.
- Creates a climate for developing future leaders.

Trust in Colleagues

Changing workplaces may experience rapid turn-around in nurse managers. More than ever, and whenever possible, **nurse**

managers should meet to mentor one another, share challenges and solutions, and have fun. Collegiality among nurse managers has several benefits, including:

- Moral support.
- Mentoring and individual or group coaching.
- Minimizing the opportunity for staff to play one practice setting off against another.

Trust in the Organization

While events associated with organizational change may challenge a nurse manager's ability to trust the workplace, each must choose to either move forward with their own measure of blind trust or go through the motions and join the ranks of the cynics and naysayers. Consider the following actions for promoting trust in your workplace:

- Take time to reflect on your own actions that inspire or inhibit trust.
- Reflect on your experience of betrayal in the workplace. Name your feelings.
- Expect people to be trustworthy and, most likely, they will be.
- Conduct a conversation with staff members about behaviors that build and betray trust. (See the discussion guide, Creating Respectful Workplace Relationships, in Appendix B).
- Lead a discussion with staff about the impact of trust on practice.

- **Invite staff to develop a Team Charter** that describes behaviors that staff commit to. Begin with, *In our workplace, we promise to. . . .*

CREATE A PLACE WHERE NURSES WANT TO WORK: TRUSTWORTHY BEHAVIORS OF SAVVY NURSE MANAGERS

The following inspiring and trust-building behaviors by nurse managers will help create a place where nurses want to work.

1. Recognize your own strengths and limitations and value the strengths of others.
2. Trust others.
3. Learn, grow, and change: Become both a teacher and a learner.
4. Lead by example: Be there (staff cannot follow if you are not present).
5. Take a leap of faith and lead into the unknown.
6. Always tell the truth.
7. Give others a chance to lead and make decisions.
8. Communicate, communicate, and, by the way communicate!
9. Own up to your mistakes.
10. Be willing to laugh at yourself.
11. Always speak positively about others.
12. Model work-life balance.

WORKPLACE CHARTERS

Developing a workplace charter is an excellent tool for reinforcing positive relationships. Some workplaces have a "code of conduct" that achieves the same end. **A workplace charter is a document developed by staff that "brings it all together": the mission, vision, values, and behaviors essential for healthy workplace relationships.** The charter is a guide for expected behaviors among staff and colleagues in their practice setting. Charters can be part of the orientation process and a tool to measure the quality of workplace relationships. Charters may include one- or two-line statements about any number of behaviors deemed important, including how decisions are made, the requirement for respect, a commitment to maintain confidentiality, expectations around meeting attendance, and conflict resolution. Typically, staff develops charters based on workplace values. Creating opportunities for conversations that will expand value statements into a workplace charter strengthens staff collegiality and minimizes feelings of powerlessness.

Fast facts in a nutshell: summary

- Meaningful practice setting mission, vision, and value statements help align staff members to a greater sense of purpose and connect them to a basic human need of contributing to the greater good.
- Charters are only relevant if they are regularly used to reinforce and guide professionalism in practice and healthy workplace relationships.

Chapter 16

Got Staff Meeting Nightmares?

Managing Awesome Opportunities

INTRODUCTION

Staff meetings are an amazing medium for transformational change. When staff groups have meaningful and positive conversations with one another, they create personal and professional power. Yet, how many times have you heard them leave a meeting and comment, "Well that was a colossal waste of time!" How do you inspire meetings so that staff members want to attend? This chapter will provide you with tips on how to structure meetings so that staff members will engage in and assume ownership for its outcomes.

In this chapter, you will learn:

1. Information about how to create conversations that matter.
2. Strategies to inspire staff from apathy to action.
3. How to manage communication at staff meetings.

TURNING AROUND THE TITANIC

Do you sometimes feel you are on a sinking ship when it comes to staff meetings? Is attendance plummeting? Scheduling a staff meeting is difficult, getting staff to attend is harder, and holding staff attention takes on nightmare proportions. In an era when time is a precious commodity, information overload is a "normal" state of affairs and demands are constant. Therefore, **staff meetings must pack a punch by being meaningful, interactive, and productive**. If you are scheduling staff meetings and no one attends, it is time to change.

Luring staff nurses from the bedside or practice setting is difficult due in part to their work ethic and the belief that meetings interfere with patient/client care. "Patient/client care" is the Number 1 reason given by staff members for not attending a meeting or leaving before it is over. While this may sometimes be true, it becomes a good excuse to avoid the pain of "nothing happening or nothing ever changes."

WHAT IF . . . THE REAL VALUE OF STAFF MEETINGS

What if staff meetings became:

- An important relational learning tool?
- A medium for personal and professional transformation?
- A vehicle for strengthening workplace relationships?
- An opportunity for nurse managers to deepen their understanding of staff relationships, identify "hot spots," or to create teachable moments?

When meetings are linked to professional development, opportunities to strengthen workplace relationships, and or improve professional practice, staff members will come.

CONSIDERATIONS FOR SCHEDULING A STAFF MEETING

The mechanics of scheduling a meeting will vary with each practice setting. The most important considerations are:

- What is the purpose of the meeting?
- How will the meeting fit with your mission and vision?
- What do you want to accomplish?
- Is there an opportunity for interactive staff learning, conversations, and/or relationship building?

PLANNING THE MEETING

A. **Develop an agenda by seeking input from staff and adding items you want to bring forward.**
B. **Define your purpose: nice to know, need to know, need your ideas.**
   1. **Nice to know: They won't attend.**
   If the meeting is an FYI only, you may want to consider another approach (i.e., a note in a communication book, e-mail, text message, or memos on the back of the bathroom door). Get creative about messaging.
   2. **Need to know: They may attend.**
   If the purpose is to share information about an issue and

receive feedback regarding the impact or their overall reactions, then schedule a meeting.

3. **Need your ideas: They will attend.**

When there is opportunity for new learning or a requirement to receive creative input from staff about how to manage a change, develop a new idea or process, or resolve an issue, staff are likely to attend.

C. **Align the purpose of the meeting with your mission and vision.**

1. **Mission matters.**

How does the meeting complement or enhance your mission. Is it an opportunity to learn about a new process to improve care or strengthen the quality of workplace relationships to enhance communication among team members? Tell the staff how the meeting furthers achievement of the mission.

2. **Value the vision.**

How will the meeting help you and your staff move toward achieving the vision for your clinical practice setting?

D. **Determine what you want to accomplish.**

Answer the question most on the minds of staff members, "What's in it for me if I attend?" They may actually get excited about attending a meeting that will be of benefit to them. The "What's in it for me?" question creates interest and peaks their curiosity.

E. **Create opportunities to learn, converse, and relate to one another.**

Build in the opportunity for discussion among and between staff members during the meeting. For example, if there is a particular issue that requires staff input, do the following:

1. Divide into smaller groups.
2. Provide each group with questions to guide their discussion.
3. Have each group record notes.
4. After 15–20 minutes, have each group provide feedback to the larger group.
5. Make notes of key points on the flipchart.
6. Develop an action plan with staff members volunteering to take responsibility for specific tasks.
7. Schedule a follow-up meeting or session.

IMPORTANT TIPS FOR GREAT STAFF MEETINGS

1. Keep them short (no longer than one hour).
2. Always have a timed agenda with staff input.
3. Make them timely (scheduling a meeting after the fact spells disaster for trustbuilding).
4. Always start and end on time.
5. Reinforce staffs' identified values to guide the meeting process.
6. Stay on topic and curb sidebars.
7. Create meaningful and timed small-group conversations and large-group feedback.
8. Use a flip chart to capture key points identified by staff.
9. Develop an action plan that staff takes responsibility for and identify a completion date.
10. In wrapping up, state the key points of the meeting and the "take-away" message(s).
11. If you have a sense of humor, use it.

12. If at all possible and if you have not already done so, try to develop your facilitation skills.

Fast facts in a nutshell

- Effective facilitation of a staff meeting ensures positive communication processes and outcomes.
- Staff meetings that are fun provide welcome relief from daily pressures, are more productive, and strengthen relationships.

OWN CONTROL: MANAGING COMMUNICATION

1. When staff members engage in sidebars, interject "I notice that some of you are having fascinating sidebar conversations. It is important to hear everyone's ideas, so I am asking that you respectfully listen to you colleagues, okay?" If this does not work, try "Yo! Listen up!"
2. Continuously scan the group for negative nonverbal communication, such as eye rolling, elbow jabbing, and sarcasm. (These behaviors require follow-up.)
3. When discussion gets off topic, try one of the following, "It appears that we are off topic. We can continue the discussion later; after the meeting; add it to the next agenda; or I can follow-up with you later." Then, get back to the topic at hand.
4. Use your knowledge of therapeutic communication techniques to reinforce staff contributions to the conversations.

5. If you are delivering "need-to-know information," capture the key points in a bulleted format to hand out to staff at the end of the meeting.
6. Conduct a "check-out" before wrap-up by asking each staff member one of the following:
   - "What is your 'take away' or 'key message' from this meeting?"
   - "What did you learn from today's meeting?"
   - "Anyone have any suggestions for how we can improve our next staff meeting?"

Fast facts in a nutshell: summary

- Regular meetings keep staff informed, promote professional practice, and relationship building
- When nurse managers facilitate successful meetings, they have the opportunity to build leadership capacity, inspire trustbuilding, and role-model excellence in communication.

Chapter 17

From Workplace to Community

Managing Connectedness

INTRODUCTION

Whether your practice setting is a nursing unit in a busy hospital, clinic, department, or outpost, you may have noticed that staff members can feel a sense of isolation or disconnectedness. It is frequently represented in the comment, "If only others knew what we really do here." How do you, as nurse manager, help individuals make connections and build new relationships within the larger organization and the community in which the healthcare setting exists? This chapter will help you help your staff bridge the organizational gaps.

In this chapter, you will learn:

1. The value of promoting staff connectedness beyond the practice setting.

2. How to encourage relationship-building capacity among staff members.
3. Tips for managing staff opportunities for connectedness.

DOWN WITH SILOS: UP WITH BUILDING RELATIONSHIPS

In addition to managing generation gaps, **Nurse Managers must also help staff build relationships by managing relationship gaps within the practice setting, the organization, and the community.** In the good ol' days, nurses tended not to focus on what was happening in the organization beyond the four walls of their practice setting. Nurses generally concerned themselves primarily with their own unit-based issues. Today, this type of thinking can be hazardous to a nurse's professional relationship health! Our relational economy requires organizations to strengthen the quality of workplace relationships to facilitate internal and external collaboration and organizational effectiveness.

THE BAD NEWS AND THE GOOD NEWS

The bad news is that many nurses now experience strong feelings of isolation and a sense of not being valued by others in the organization. These feelings may shed light on the powerlessness that so often accompanies the victims of organizational change or reflect oppressed group behavior.

The good news is that today, through a slow process of osmosis, **nurses are learning more about the work of the or-**

ganization, how their practice setting complements that work, and the overall organizational impact on the well-being of the communities in which they serve.

Cross-pollination is occurring, as nurses participate with other staff members on organizational committees. In-patient nurses are teaching in the community. In a variety of practice settings, staff members are conducting "open houses" to showcase their work. The better news is that, for the most part, nurses love it! Despite the disgruntled comments from a few negaholics, nurses' professional worlds are expanding in their influence in healthcare. Furthermore, others are seeing the value that nurses bring to the organizational table, the community, and beyond.

A BLESSING AND A CURSE

Almost everything has an up side and down side. When inspiring staff members to spread their organizational wings into domains once considered exclusive to the nurse manager's responsibilities, staff nurses are conducting conversations and making decisions that extend beyond their practice setting. This can be both a blessing and a curse. On one hand, nurses may enhance relationship building. However, taking nurses beyond their comfort zone may require some nurse managers to engage in "damage control." Consider this a natural part of the learning process, one in which you are willing to extend trust and consider mistakes as opportunities to learn. The purpose is to facilitate professional development. The benefits of facilitating relational learning opportunities for nurses include:

- Broadening nurses' individual and collective professional perspectives.
- Building leadership capacity as nurses represent their practice settings.
- Creating opportunities for expanding nurses' organizational learning regarding the culture, politics, and relationships that influence the healthcare setting.
- Facilitating two-way communication between frontline staff, the organization, and community, and vice versa.
- Increasing nurses' autonomy through direct involvement in decision making.
- Positioning nurses to positively influence professional practice organization wide and beyond.

Fast facts in a nutshell

- Facilitating connectedness creates opportunities for personal and professional growth through new learning, new conversations, and new experiences that promote excellence in practice and positive quality of work life.
- The process of connectedness and strengthening relationships begins when nurse managers move out of the comfort zone of their practice setting, get involved and become more visible across and beyond the organization.

INFLUENCING CONNECTEDNESS: CONDUCT A SELF-AWARENESS CHECK

- How connected are you to the larger organization? Do you lead, follow, or get out of the way? Are you a Lemming or an "organizational maverick"?
- Do you participate in, speak up, initiate, or lead the introduction of innovative ideas at the organizational level?
- What profile do you have in the community?
- Staff members are likely to follow your lead. If you are not connected, then it will be difficult to inspire your staff. On the other hand, if you are too connected and spend most of your time away from the practice setting, staff members may resent your absence and resist your efforts to involve them.

MANAGING THE BALANCE CHALLENGE OF CONNECTEDNESS

Learning to broaden your connections while maintaining stability in your practice setting is a delicate balance. Consider it as an art form and a work in process. Where, when, and how you make connections beyond your workplace comes with trial and error. It also depends on the level of professional autonomy among your staff members and your own comfort level.

Trial and Error

In attempting to broaden your connections and model connectedness, it is easy to become overinvolved in external committee work, projects, and planning exercises. Be prepared to step back if staff members begin to complain that you are "never there." In their heads, they are saying, "There's no way I'm spending my time away from my patients working on committees, I'll never have time be with my patients."

Level of Professional Autonomy Among Staff

When your staff possesses a high level of professional autonomy, you may be able to spend more time away from your workplace to advance your connectedness, spread your professional influence, and demonstrate formal leadership at a higher level.

When staff members have less professional autonomy and require more supervision, coaching, and role modeling, they have a higher need for your visible presence. This may require you to pick and choose your connection opportunities according to your availability. For example, your practice setting may be less hectic in the afternoon, thereby freeing you up for committee participation.

Your Comfort Level

Severing the proverbial umbilical cord by breaking away from your practice setting and forging new relationship in advancing professional connectedness may feel uncomfortable at first, and you may want to retreat to your familiar turf.

- Resist the urge to run and run hard! It will get better.
- Give yourself permission to feel your way along as you journey down this new road. This is not unlike the feeling you may have had as a new mother leaving your child with the babysitter for the first time.
- Help staff members to understand your absence by reporting to them about what you are doing, what you are learning, and how your involvement benefits their practice.

TIPS FOR MANAGING STAFF OPPORTUNITIES FOR PROMOTING RELATIONSHIP-BUILDING CONNECTEDNESS

There are countless opportunities for connecting beyond your workplace that include:

1. Modeling connecting behaviors, such as becoming an "in-house" speaker on specific topics, inviting staff in the organization to come and see the work of your practice setting, writing an article, leading an initiative, asking members of the community to participate on a practice setting committee.
2. Supporting opportunities for staff to lead initiatives that may impact the organization, such as time off for participation on committees
3. Facilitating conversations about the value of staff connecting beyond the practice setting.

4. Educating staff members about your committee involvement by taking them to a meeting (this depends of course on the nature of the committee meeting, prior approval and support from the committee as a whole).
5. Encouraging and supporting staff to conduct an "open house."
6. Encouraging and providing time for staff members to write about their practice for publication in a professional journal or an organizational newsletter.
7. Encouraging them to invite staff from other departments to your workplace to talk about how they can support one another or strengthen their working relationships.
8. Meeting with individual nurses to talk about their aspirations for influencing practice beyond the level of their practice setting. (Some at first may have no desire whatsoever. Keep an eye on this attitude as a developmental opportunity for your future attention.)
9. Creating structures for staff members to provide feedback on their off-unit professional activities.
10. Providing opportunities for leadership development within the practice setting, such as team leading, chairing the occasional staff meeting, clinical teaching, attending nursing practice development meetings, or taking a staff nurse with you to meet with another department representative.
11. Advocating for staff nurse representation on committees that would not normally even consider their presence.
12. Inviting staff to participate in presentations to senior leadership
13. Looking for opportunities in the community for staff nurses to "strut their stuff," as, for example, health teach-

ing in schools, facilitating focus groups, running for political office, participating in career days, and attending and presenting at conferences on local, national, and international levels.

14. Coaching or facilitating the acquisition of resources to support the nurses' ability to speak up and speak out.

Connectedness is the foundation of excellence in nursing practice. Nurse managers must lead the way in extending this competency beyond the bedside and practice settings.

Part V

From Surviving to Thriving
Tips and Tools for Thriving
in a Changing Workplace

Chapter 18

Top Ten Fast Facts for Thriving in a Changing Workplace

Twelve More for Managing It!

INTRODUCTION

Thriving in a changing workplace does not happen by chance. In a thriving workplace, nurse managers possess high levels of self-awareness, set the tone for excellence in practice, and require values-driven healthy workplace relationships to achieve a healing environment and therapeutic practice setting. When nurse managers thrive, so does the staff. The following Top Ten Fast Facts lists key strategies for thriving, as opposed to just surviving, on a personal and managerial level.

In this chapter, you will learn:

1. Top ten **personal** tips for thriving in a changing workplace.
2. Top twelve **management** tips for creating a thriving workplace.

TOP TEN PERSONAL TIPS FOR THRIVING IN A CHANGING WORKPLACE

1. **Choose your attitude wisely.**
You have the power to choose your attitude. **When you choose a positive attitude you change the quality of your future.**
2. **Take care of yourself.**
If you do not take care of yourself, who will? You cannot adequately lead and manage a thriving workplace and create a happy home life if you do not have balance. Get help if you need it. You are after all, only human! Start small by taking relaxing baths and slowly build up to Mediterranean cruises!
3. **Get your priorities straight.**
At the end of the day, what really matters most? Reflect on your values and determine if your personal values match your workplace values.
4. **Pick your battles; you can't win them all.**
Ask yourself, "Is this the hill I want to die on?" Try to identify what you can control and/or influence. If you cannot do either, move on.
5. **Remember the three R's: respect for self, respect for others, and respect for your organization.**
Reflect on R-E-S-P-E-C-T. Do you require being treated with respect? How respectful are you of others?
6. **Focus on today; yesterday is history; tomorrow is a mystery.**
Today is all that you have.
7. **"Be the change you wish to see" (Gandhi) and inspire it in others.**
Walk the talk; do what you say you will; treat others the way you wish to be treated. Live your values!

8. **The best way to predict your future is to create it.**
Determine what you want in your future, and then set about to create it!

9. **Cultivate or resurrect your sense of humor.**
Well-placed humor is both infectious and therapeutic. If you have a sense of humour, use it. If you do not, that's okay too. Appropriate laughter in the workplace becomes conspicuous by its absence. When staff members say, "We never laugh here anymore," it is time to find ways to lighten up. Grab a teaspoon and prepare to administer a dose of levity. After all, laughter is good medicine!

10. **Don't wait for others to change; you go first!**
If you are holding your breath waiting for someone else to change their behavior; two things will happen:

1. They will not change, and . . .
2. You will turn blue!

TOP TWELVE MANAGEMENT TIPS FOR THRIVING IN A CHANGING WORKPLACE

1. **Always tell the truth.**
Staff members know when you are not being upfront and will "fill in the blanks" with what *they think* is missing. Before you know it, the grist for the organizational rumour mill is churned out at warp speed.

2. **Authentic leaders have nothing to hide.**
They inspire trust

3. **Expect respect for all.**
Require respectful behavior from and toward all staff members, physicians, patients, families, and visitors.

4. In crises, look for opportunities; in opportunities, expect snags!

Most change can create reactions ranging from the good to the bad to the ugly. Snags may be blessings in disguise. Look for the possibilities.

6. Create a place where staff wants to work!

Creating a practice environment grounded in excellence begins with you. You set the tone, you hire the right staff, you communicate expectations, you inspire staff through regular feedback and you challenge them to soar both personally and professionally.

7. Create opportunities for fascinating group conversations, inspired dialogue, and possibilities!

Staff meetings are one of the most powerful tools for a nurse manager. Craft agendas that excite, energize, and invite conversations and laughter. Then, staff will attend! If you supply refreshments, staff will beat down the door!

8. Breathe life into the Standards of Practice.

When staff performance deviates from the Standards of Practice and members are not held accountable, they start on a slippery professional slope that can negatively affect the quality of care and worklife. You cannot monitor adherence to the Standards if you are not present in the practice setting to draw attention to them! If you are present, you can assess staff's competence, identify their learning needs, and determine where they fit on the professional practice autonomy scale.

9. Build your workplace mission, vision, and values to guide professional practice and quality of worklife.

Staff members do well when they are confident that there is a good organizational fit between their skills and the required work. They also need to know how their workplace fits into the context of the organization, as well as the guidelines and actions that govern behaviors to accomplish what needs to be done. A practice setting mission, vision, and values statement is a compass that gives direction to the workplace and all who work there.

10. **Deal with unacceptable behavior by reinforcing professionalism at all times and practicing performance management.**

Although one of the most uncomfortable processes that nurse managers must face, dealing with untoward behavior is never optional. The longer the behavior goes unchecked, the greater the potential for destroying workplace relationships essential to professional practice, staff well-being, and quality of care.

11. **You cannot be a friend to staff and manage them at the same time.**

Being a friend to staff is a boundary issue about meeting your needs and not about meeting staff needs.

12. **Facilitate self-directed learning, listen to what is not being said, and encourage solution-focused conversations.**

Fast facts in a nutshell: summary

Thriving in a changing workplace requires you to give yourself three gifts:
- The gift of time to reflect.
- The gift of a positive attitude.
- The gift of courage to create your future.

Discussion Guides
Tools to Inspire Creative Conversations

The discussion guides presented below can be used to inspire conversations, ignite creativity, and promote staff engagement in initiating and/or managing change.

Feel free to adapt these tools to fit your situation. When staff members follow the guidelines and write down comments based on their conversations, the written word takes on greater significance. This recorded conversation can then serve as a point of reference to create action plans and benchmarks for evaluation of staff initiatives.

The guides are:

Appendix A

Postcard from Home

PURPOSE

This exercise helps staff MEMBERS identify what they believe to be the ideal work environment. From this you can extract a mission, vision, and values statement for your practice setting.

1. Divide staff into groups of 3.
2. Ask them to pretend that they have a friend working in another country and they want the friend to consider returning home to work in your practice setting. Ask staff to complete the following:

Dear _____

I am writing to you to entice you to return home to work in our practice setting _____. I believe that this is the most professionally fulfilling workplace that I have ever worked in because:

Please give it some thought.

Have each group read their cards to the whole group. Look for common threads between the groups and their content. Ask for volunteers to collect the postcards and prepare a draft for the remaining staff to critique. Revise again until staff agrees with the revisions.

Appendix B

Creating Respectful
Workplace Relationships

One issue in workplace relationships is living the value of
respect. *

1. It is important to address this issue because:

2. We all have a role to play in creating healthy and respect-
    ful workplace relationships. We believe that:

A. Individuals could demonstrate respect by doing the fol-
    lowing:

B. Managers could demonstrate respect by doing the following:

C. Staff could demonstrate respect by doing the following:

D. As a whole, the organization could demonstrate that all
    relationships are founded on the value of respect by:

E. Union and Management could together demonstrate re-
    spectful relationships when they:

*Substitute any value such as: accountability; compassion; excellence; col-
laboration etc.

Appendix C

Living Our Values Discussion Guide

Our workplace value of _____
(use words like accountability, compassion, excellence, respect, and caring).

In our practice setting we believe that *accountability* is essential. We define accountability as: _____

1. Staff will know that they are being accountable when they:

2. Patients, clients, and their families will see that staff is ac-
    countable when:

3. Other colleagues will know that we are accountable as a
    staff group when:

Appendix D

Back to Our Future Exercise

PART 1   PURPOSE

This powerful and creative exercise allows groups of staff to intermingle and collaborate in a fun way. It is designed to "get them on the same page," allow "baggage" to surface in a non-threatening way, and to share ideas.

Equipment

1 flip chart page per table group
1 box of crayons

1. Where were we (in the good ol' days)?	2. Where we are now?
3. Where do we want to be?	4. How are we going to get there?

Instructions

1. Instruct the groups to divide the flip chart page into four sections, with each quadrant labeled as seen above.
2. Groups are then asked to draw with crayons their responses to the headings.
3. Rules for artwork: No people or stick figures allowed. Words are to be kept to a minimum. Animals, birds, insects, flowers, objects, and anything else nonhuman are allowed. Have fun! No spying between groups!

Process

1. Allow 20 to 30 minutes to complete artwork.
2. Observe the group dynamics and the laughter!

3. Invite people to the front of the room to explain their pictures.
4. After everyone has presented, ask the following questions:
   A. In your table group: What did you hear? What did you see? What did you learn?
   B. In the large group: What did you hear in your group? What did you see? What did you learn?

The lessons this exercise teaches include:

In **Quadrant # 1**: Initially, staff glorifies the good ol' days, but then realizes maybe that is not correct.

In **Quadrant # 2**: Staff sees that today's workplace relationships are a mixture of strengths and needs for improvement. They recognize that most people want to make things work.

In **Quadrant # 3**: The pictures usually depict a workplace utopia where staff is happy and relaxed. Themes of vacationers on a Caribbean island, ants, and geese flying in unison are usually depicted.

In **Quadrant # 4**: Pictures include hands together, hearts, collaboration, technology, money, etc.

KEY MESSAGES FROM THIS EXERCISE

Following the large group discussion, summarize the following key messages:

1. Respect for diversity: despite their differences, they achieved their goal.

2. No one has all the answers: Together they are better.
2. Results oriented: Ability to complete the task in a relatively short period of time.
3. Laughter: Because of the sound of laughter was so obvious, the task went much easier. Staff members still had the ability to laugh and having fun at work is not only okay, it is doable!
4. Creativity: Staff members discovers that working together generates creativity.
5. Collaboration: People listened.

Appendix E

Back to the Future Discussion Guide

INSTRUCTIONS

Once staff have completed the artwork exercise, instruct them to think about Quadrants # 3 and 4 and complete this discussion guide. For us to adapt to our changing workplaces and create our futures, each of us will have to learn, grow, and change.

Some things that we may have to learn include:

1.
2.
3.

Things that will help us to grow personally and professionally include:

1.
2.
3.

Strategies that we can use as individuals to help each other to manage change could include:

1.
2.
3.

Our Nurse Manager can help us manage change by:

One suggestion for the union to help members manage change would be to:

Appendix F

Creating Our Values

PURPOSE

To help staff members develop values that will govern their workplace relationships.

EQUIPMENT

Flip chart at front of room; 1 flip chart page for each group; and 1 piece of paper for each person

INSTRUCTIONS

1. Ask staff to form small groups of 3 to 4 people.
2. As you stand in next to a flip chart, ask staff members to call out one-word values that they believe to be important in the workplace. Write them down in list format on the flip chart (no more than 15).
3. Ask each person to pick five that he or she feels is most important, write them down on a piece of paper, and then

discuss his or her choices in the small groups. Have one person in each group record all the choices in a list on one page. Where the values are repeated, make a check mark next to the value.

4. Each small group then selects their top three, which are recorded on your flip chart to create a list. Look for duplicates.

5. Create a new consolidated list and ask each staff person to come forward and check off her/his three top values. Select the three or four values that received the most checkmarks.

REFERENCES

Barker, J. (1988). *Discover the future: The business of paradigms.* St. Paul: ILI Press

Beer, M., & Eisenstat, R. (2000). The silent killers of strategy implementation and learning. *Sloan Management Review, 41*(4), 29–40.

Bennis, W. (1997). *Managing people is like herding cats.* Provo, UT: Executive Excellence Publishing.

Bridges, W. (1991). *Managing transitions: Making the most of change.* Reading, MA: Perseus Books.

Drucker, P. (1989). The new realities. New York: Harper & Rowe. In E. Oakley & D. Krug, (1991). Enlightened leadership: Getting to the heart of change. (p. 191). New York: Simon & Schuster.

Fisher, H. (1999). *The first sex: The natural talents of women and how they are changing the world.* New York: Random House.

Freire, P. (1997). *Pedagogy of the oppressed.* New York: Continuum.

Fry, B. (2003). Facilitating workplace relational learning. The intersection of power, caring and quality of worklife.

Masters thesis. St. Francis Xavier University. Antigonish, Nova Scotia, Canada.

Government of Canada, Work/life balance and new workplace challenges: Frequently asked questions." Retrieved 6/15/2006 from http:www.canadian-network.ca

Hankin, H. (2005). *The new workforce: five sweeping trendsthat will shape your company's future.* New York: AMACOM

Hutchinson, M., Jackson, D., Vickers, M., and Wilkes, L. (2006). Workplace bullying in nursing: Towards a more critical organizational perspective. Abstract from *Nursing Inquiry, 13,* 118–126. Retrieved from the internet 09/02/07.

Kupperschmidt, B. (2000). Multi-generation employees: Strategies for effective management. *Health Care Management 19,* 65–76.

Marshall, E. (1995). *Transforming the way we work.* New York: AMACOM.

Maurer, R. (1996). *Beyond the wall of resistance.* Austin, TX: Bard

Nazarko, L. (2000). Bullying and harassment. *Nursing Management, 8*(1), 14–16.

Oakley, E., & Krug, D. (1994). *Enlightened Leadership: getting to the heart of change.* New York: Simon & Schuster.

Peplau, H. (1988). *Interpersonal relations in nursing.* London: MacMillan Education.

Reina, D., & Reina, M. (2006). *Trust and betrayal in the workplace: Building effective relationships in your organization* (pp. 128–140). Berret-Kohler: San Francisco.

Roberts, S. J. (1983). Oppressed group behavior: Implications for nursing. *Advances in Nursing Science, 5*(3), 21–30.

Roberts, S. (2000). Development of a positive identity: Liberating oneself from the oppressor within. *Advances in Nursing Science, 22*(4), 71–82.

Russell, S., & Shirk, B. (1993). Women's anger and eating. In S. P. Thomas (Ed.), *Women and anger* (pp. 170–185). New York: Springer.

Short, R. (1998). *Learning in relationship: Foundations for personal and professional success.* Bellevue, WA: Learning Technologies.

Sullivan, E. (2004). *Becoming influential: A guide for nurses.* Upper Saddle River, NJ: Pearson Prentice Hall

Thomas, S., Smucker, C., & Droppleman, P. (1998). It hurts most around the heart: A phenomenological exploration of women's anger. *Journal of Advanced Nursing, 28*(2), 311–322.

Thomas, S. (1993). *Women and anger.* New York: Springer Publishing.

Thomas, S. (2004). *Transforming nurses' stress and anger; Steps toward healing anger* (pp15–32). New York: Springer.

Thomas, S., & Jefferson, C. (1996). *Use your anger; A woman's guide to empowerment.* New York: Pocket Books.

Tulgan, B. (2002). *Winning the talent wars: How to build a lean, flexible, high-performance workplace.* London: Norton.

Vaill, P. (1996). *Learning as a way of being: Strategies for survival in a world of permanent white water.* San Francisco: Jossey-Bass.

Index